# A Desperate Need

## A Guide to Treating Addictions and Recapturing Life

Stephen L. Hufman MD

Cover photograph by Stephen L. Hufman
Published in Leavenworth, WA by To Serve and Encourage Publications
Visit authors website: stephenhufman.com.



ISBN: 978-1-7336456-0-7 (paperback)
ISBN: 978-1-7336456-1-4 (ebk)

# Table of Contents

# Introduction

These pages do not contain a secret formula for curing addictions as no one has discovered the panacea for drug abuse. Neither is this an attempt to replace drug treatment centers, whose varied approaches range from expensive retreat spas for the rich and famous to street corner methadone clinics. All have some success, but all unfortunately have many failures. The major problem for most people is that a qualified, affordable program is not available in their area. This is a travesty that our nation is only beginning to wake up to.

> Of the 24.6 million people addicted to drugs or alcohol, roughly only 1 in 10 will get any treatment. Even then the treatment is usually one time only.

However, the other major problem I see is that many treatment programs are unable to treat the entire range of the disease because their approach downplays the spiritual/emotional aspect of addictions and does not fully recognize the need for healing of the spirit. This book is an attempt to help people develop their own program with the resources available to them and begin on the road to recovery.

People are dying each day from drug overdose, and many more struggle with addictions that rob them of home, family, and a future. This book is an attempt to provide people with practical tools to start them on the road to recovery. My hope is to help those suffering with addictions, along with their family and friends. I desire to help them find a way out of the darkness of this terrible curse and into the light of life. It all begins with realizing we have a desperate need for healing, and a God who wants to meet our need and heal us. This, combined with a steadfast support from people willing to let God direct their help, can ultimately break the chains of addiction.

Remember, this is a curse that is ruining lives. Our goal

SECTION 1

# Recognizing the Desperate Need

*"The heart is deceitful above all things and beyond cure. Who can understand it?" Jeremiah 17:9*

There is no possibility of change without acceptance of the need for change.

CHAPTER 1

# A Terrible Deception

"Doc, what am I supposed to do? You gotta help me."

My patient and good friend, Bill, pleaded with me for another Percocet prescription (oxycodone with Tylenol).

"This back pain won't let me sit in a forklift all day. How am I going to feed my family? You've got to give me something Doc. How about some Oxys just to make it through my shift; I won't use them otherwise."

He stared at me with large black pupils begging for help, his hands trembling uncontrollably, beads of sweat on his forehead. I felt unsure of what to do next and prayed for wisdom.

"Bill, I think you're going through opiate withdrawal," I said. "We need to get you into a drug treatment program, not give you more opiates."

"I'm no druggie, Doc. You know that. Besides, who's going to pay for it? I can't put bread on the table from some hospital."

Some signs of opiate withdrawal:

Depression, Anxiety, Insomnia, Vomiting

Diarrhea, Abdominal cramps,

Sweating, Muscle, bone, and joint aches

Loss of appetite, Runny nose

Dilated pupils

My mind searched for answers I didn't have. We lived in a small isolated town over 160 miles to the next major city. The local twenty bed hospital barely covered medical problems, surgeries and deliveries, we were definitely not prepared to handle acute drug withdrawal.

In people using prescription opiates for chronic pain, 8 - 12 percent will go on to develop an addiction. These prescription opiates include: codeine, hydrocodone (Vicodin), oxycodone (Percocet / Percodan), meperidine (Demerol), hydromorphone (Dilaudid), methadone, fentanyl (Duragesic), and morphine. Suboxone (Buprenorphine) is not an opiate but is prescribed to prevent withdrawal as an addiction treatment drug.

"Doc, you're the one who gave me the pain killers for my back in the first place. You can't just cut me off now!"

Bill had a point; eight months ago I had first seen him for lumbar strain. We both figured it would go away with time and physical therapy. To allow him to work during this period, I gave him some Vicodin. He promised to only take it for emergencies. Pretty soon he began taking them on a regular basis to keep working. After a few months the Vicodin seemed to lose its potency, so I switched him to the stronger Percocet, just to make work tolerable.

Accommodation (or tolerance) occurs in most people after 4-6 weeks of opiate use. This means the initial dose no longer produces the desired effect. Dose increases are common. Two serious problems occur with accommodation: 1. Higher doses take one closer to the lethal dose, increasing the risk of death, and 2. Abstaining for a period may decrease your tolerance to the drug causing accidental overdose with previously tolerated drug amount.

"I'll give you just enough for three weeks, but, we have to come up with a plan to get you off narcotics by the next visit." I started writing out a prescription conflicted about what would really help.

Bill showed up unexpected at the clinic two days before his scheduled follow-up appointment.

"Sorry I am here a bit early, but I am going on a weekend hunting trip and won't be here for my appointment. I figured you'd understand."

"I thought we were going to discuss a plan for getting off these?" I said with some concern. "I can't drop everything to get into this right now; there are other patients I have to see."

"It's okay Doc, we can talk that all out next time. Besides my friend is waiting for me outside. Oh, and could you make it for a few extra? I don't want to mess up the hunting trip with back pain."

Feeling uneasy, but not wanting to get behind, I caved in to Bill's request. "Make sure you cancel your appointment and make another. How many do you need?"

"Same as last time and ten for hunting."

Bill watched as I reluctantly wrote out the prescription. I tore it off the pad and handed it to him with the instructions: "Tell the receptionist we'll need extra time to work on the plan. No more mess ups; I won't be making any more allowances."

"You bet, Doc." Bill left the office without looking back.

A few weeks later, Bill came in two days before his scheduled appointment. The nurse caught me between patients.

"He insisted he had to see you so I put him in the procedure room," she said with a shrug. "He seems a little more jumpy than usual."

Upon entering the room, Bill started right in talking. "Doc, I think the pharmacy shorted me last time. Can you give me some more?... Just enough till our appointment."

"Bill, you're giving me the run-around. I think you're going through your pills a lot faster than I prescribed."

"Well, I can't sit in that forklift without something, and I only take them when I need them. If you won't give me some, you'll be forcing me to get them some other way. I have to work or I'll lose my pickup and then my house. You just can't do this to my family!"

It struck me as ironic that our town was too small for drug treatment, but large enough to get whatever you wanted off the street. "Bill, I can't keep giving you narcotics. I think you need to enter rehab." I was tired of this game of constantly trying to figure out the truth about Bill's drug use.

"Don't make me feel like some drug addict! You're the one who gave them to me in the first place."

I shook my head. "I'm afraid we are not getting any closer to getting you off these narcotics. I can't keep doing this. It's not helping you, or right for me."

"I just need enough to make it to my vacation next month, then I'll use those two weeks to come off of them. I promise," Bill pleaded.

I considered this request, Bill seemed sincere. "Okay, but you have to agree not to take more than what's stated on the label."

"You bet, Doc." Bill's voice settled back into his normal friendly tone.

"So how many do you need?" My pen poised over the prescription pad.

Bill quickly responded, "One hundred and thirty; that should cover the next two weeks, and one refill will get me to my vacation."

"Wow, that's more than eight per day," I exclaimed doing a quick calibration in my head. "You're going to have liver problems. I only want you to take seven per day at the maximum, and be careful you don't get acetaminophen from other sources."

"Sure. Anything you say, Doc," Bill reassured me.

Tylenol or acetaminophen can cause liver damage at doses above 4,000 mg per day in adults. Because it is a common ingredient in many over-the-counter medications a person can easily exceed this amount and not realize it.

"Let's see… fourteen-day supply at seven per day equals ninety-eight pills… I'll give you an even one hundred. That should last you until Friday two weeks from today with two left over."

"What about a refill to get me to my vacation?"

"No, I need to see you and make sure things are going all right."

"Whatever Doc, you're the one in charge. I'll see you in two weeks." He shook my hand, grabbed the prescription, and raced out the door.

~

The first obstacle for most people involved with addictions is denial. The mind uses it as a protective measure to avoid facing uncomfortable truths. In addictions, it allows the person to block out the shame of what enslaves them. No one wants to face the painful truth of what has happened. When the person is in denial about their addiction or codependency, they rebuff any attempt by others to help them recover because they fear having their personal shame exposed and/or lose their only coping mechanism. Accountability groups can help by members being transparent about their own struggles and demonstrating the transforming power of the God's Spirit. Then, with compassion they can come alongside and remind the person of the real hope we all share in Jesus.

Israel had a strong problem of denial:

*"When people fall down, don't they get up again? When they discover they're on the wrong road, don't they turn back? Then why do these people stay on their self-destructive path? Why do the people of Jerusalem refuse to turn back? They cling tightly to their lies and will not turn around." Jeremiah 8:4-5 NLT*

Part of Israel's deception centered on treating the problem as a superficial cut rather than a mortal wound. In their minds they rationalized, "It's not that bad."

*"They offer superficial treatments for my people's mortal wound. They give assurances of peace when there is no peace." Jeremiah 8:11 NLT*

God understood that Israelites did not have the strength or ability to save themselves, but He loved them too much to let go. So, the Lord reveals His plan to send a Great Physician to heal and offer hope of a new life.

*"But when the teachers of religious law who were Pharisees saw him eating with tax collectors and other sinners, they asked his disciples, 'Why does he eat with such scum?'*
*When Jesus heard this, he told them, 'Healthy people don't need a doctor—sick people do. I have come to call not those who think they are righteous, but those who know they are sinners.'" Mark 2:16-17 NLT*

Denial can be hard to break through, but trusting in God, His mercy and compassion, offers us real hope in Jesus. Our role is to follow in His steps.

CHAPTER 2

# Caught Up in a Lie

At the appointment on Friday, the eve of Bill's vacation, I thought I could easily deal with his problem. Just slowly taper him down over ten days to avoid severe withdrawal, then he would be off.

"I'll give you one less each day over the next seven days plus two in case there is a problem. That's a total of 30 pills. I want to see you in a week to make sure things are going as planned."

Bill took the prescription and left without a word.

Looking back, I am chagrined at my own naiveté. I had no idea of the power of addictions and Bill's desperate need for help.

A little later after the office had closed, I received a call from the pharmacist.

"Did you know I just filled a prescription for Bill from Dr. Burns for sixty Oxycodone a week ago?" asked the pharmacist.

"What? Bill didn't even tell me he was seeing another doctor," I said.

"It appears Bill has been using two pharmacies as well," the pharmacist continued. "I called Hometown Drug, and they have been filling your scripts unaware of Dr. Burn's prescriptions for Percodan being filled here. It appears Bill forgot which pharmacy he used for which doctor."

"How long has this been going on?"

"About three months."

"Three months!" I was in shock. "I can't believe Bill would do this."

"Do you want me to fill your prescription?"

"No. Void it. And tell him I need to see him. I'll call Dr. Burns and we'll come up with a plan."

As I hung up, feelings of betrayal and anger surged. *How could my friend lie to me like this? Use me! We go to church together. I trusted him like a brother.*

As I struggled with being deceived, I realized I had no answers as to what to do next; I could only wait for Bill to return and confront him with the truth.

Thankfully, I didn't see Bill at church that Sunday. I could not discuss it out of the office, and seeing him at church would have made for a very awkward moment.

Addictions make a person lie and cheat, but the person lied to and cheated the most is themselves. Honesty is hard for addicts, for then they have to face the truth of their problem.

On Monday, Bill called, and we squeezed him in at 4:30 at the end of the schedule. I spent the day thinking about that appointment and what I would say without getting angry.

He showed up in the reception area just before five, with his two young children in tow.

"Sorry I am late," he told the receptionist. "I had to watch the kids after work and it took me longer than I expected to get them ready and in the car. I hope you don't mind me bringing them, but I really had no choice."

My nurse checked him in and put them all in the exam room. I excused the staff to leave for the day since I had no idea how long this would take. As I opened the exam room door, I said a quick prayer for guidance and went in.

Bill sat bouncing his two-year-old daughter, Lindsey, on his knee trying to keep her entertained while his son Davy had laid face down on my stool, spinning himself like a top.

"Doc, I am sorry about the mix-up. I should have told you, but I needed to make sure I had enough medication to make it through the first two days of my vacation. My wife just found out she has to work extra shifts, and I didn't want to be watching the kids and going through withdrawal. I'm sure you understand my dilemma."

"But you had obtained multiple prescriptions over the last three months from Dr. Burns," I countered. "Your story doesn't add up. I think you're not telling me the whole truth." It took all my effort to remain calm.

"Daddy, I'm tired, can we go home now?" Davy looked up from the stool at his father.

Bill put his hand on Davy, "We'll be going as soon as I am finished talking with the doctor." He switched his gaze to me. "I have to be a dad to my kids and it's harder on my back than sitting in the forklift. What are you going to do when your kids run and jump in your arms? They don't understand about back pain when they want to play horsey. So you tell me, Doc. What am I supposed to do?"

"There is not going to be an easy solution, Bill, but let's start with you being honest with me. How many pills per day are you taking?"

"I just take them when I need them, sometimes I just take a half. I don't keep track." He shifted in his chair and bounced Lindsey a little more.

"Do you have any left?"

"No, I ran out yesterday, since you canceled my prescription. That's why I wasn't at church."

"I'm confused," I said trying to sort out just how much Bill had been taking. "Give me an approximate number per day."

"Oh, eight or nine, maybe." Bill said looking at his daughter who began to squirm wanting to get down.

Davy started opening drawers on the exam table. I stepped in front to keep him from getting into the speculums.

"Davy, close that, and get over here!" Bill yelled.

"This doesn't add up to the number of pills you have received in the past month from Dr. Burns and me. You should have plenty left." I said barely controlling my anger.

Bill grabbed his son by the arm whereupon Davy squealed and sat down to resist. Lindsey wiggled in his other arm, trying to join her brother on the floor.

"Well, some fell into the toilet because when I have pain I get the shakes and I spilled them," Bill explained. "The pain is killing me. I gotta work… Doc you gotta help me, just this time… at least for my family!"

"Daaaddy, I'm hungry," Davy whined.

"The back pain is not going to kill you," I said. "But I do know if you continue like you have been, this opiate addiction will destroy you and your family. You have escalated the use of Oxycodone and Tylenol, putting yourself at risk of overdosing. You're building a tolerance to these pain killers and you have to continue upping the dose to achieve any pain relief. One day, you'll nod off while driving and have an accident, or just never wake up. Then what's your family going to do?"

"Oh, Doc, that's not going to happen! I'll be real careful, I promise." Bill said, trying to control his children.

"You've been lying to me these past few weeks; how do I know you're not lying now?" I challenged.

"Doc, you never asked if I had gotten any Oxys from Dr. Burns. I am telling you the truth. Please, you have to believe me."

"Daddy, let's go," Davy twisted his arm, trying to free himself.

"Daddy's almost done, it won't be too much longer." Bill's eyes pleaded with me to give him a break.

"You know Bill, the biggest lie you are telling is the one you're telling yourself," I said sadly.

"Daddy, I need to go pee." Davy started to escalate his volume.

I continued, "Bill, I won't leave you hanging; I helped create this monster, but you have to work with me. No more lying, half-truths, or not telling the whole story."

"Daaaddyyy!" Hollered Davy.

Suddenly, a sound came from Lindsey's diaper.

"Your in charge, Doc, you control the Oxys," Bill said. Another stinky phaaaat came from Lindsey. "Sorry, do you have a diaper I could borrow? I forgot the diaper bag."

I paused, then started to laugh. "Not exactly the apology I had hoped for," I said, pulling a diaper from the shelf. "But we all have a desperate need, so I guess we'll start from here."

As Bill began to change Lindsey on the exam table, I took Davy to the bathroom. When we returned, I got out my prescription pad.

"Now tell me again, how many pills are you using a day? I'm switching you to straight oxycodone without Tylenol to avoid hurting your liver."

"I need ten a day of the 10 milligram tablets."

I tried unsuccessfully to hide my shock.

"You told me to be honest," said Bill, packing up the kids to leave.

I held the office door open as he shuffled out and remarked to Bill, "I know taking care of your children is important, but bringing them to your appointment and coming in late makes it difficult for us to focus and deal with your addiction. Occasionally emergencies arise and it cannot be helped, but in the future, I want you to plan ahead and come alone and on time."

"Doc, do you think I intentionally..."

"Daddy, come on!"

~

Bill used his children and coming in late as a means to engender sympathy from me and get a prescription without having to face the hard task of getting off opiates. A major red flag in substance abuse is lying, or offering only half the truth. This is how the addict will try to avoid facing the truth about themselves. Consequently, this is one of the first steps in recovery—a sincere commitment to being honest; to living the truth.

You can't make the right choices or get help when you are lying to yourself and others about your plight. Who will seek help when they don't think they have a serious problem? True honesty in addictions requires swallowing your pride, and admitting you are enslaved to drugs and can't control it. But isn't that how confession is for all of us—a stripping away of any pretense about who we are so that the Lord can forgive us… and help us… and give us hope in our desperate need?

Some signs of manipulation:

Lying or omitting parts of the truth.
Denying or rationalizing responsibility.
Using anger to divert attention.
Playing the victim.
Minimizing their actions ("boys will be boys," or "the devil made me do it").
Intimidation.
Diversion.
Laying on a guilt trip ("If you hadn't been so ___").
Shame (redirect attention to another person's shortcomings).

CHAPTER 3

# A Problem of Pride

In two weeks, Bill returned to the office for a refill of his oxycodone and to discuss the taper.

"So how did it go?" I asked.

"Fine," replied Bill in a flat voice.

"That's nice." Sensing a problem, I probed further, "How many pills do you have left?"

"None."

"You should have three left for the rest of this day," I said trying not to sound accusatory.

Bill began to fidget and avoided making eye contact.

"Well, I may have taken a few extra on really tough days," he said with a shrug.

"Bill, you are not being honest with me. If you are not going to be totally truthful, we are wasting our time. I sense there is a wall between us, and it has to do with what you are not telling me. Now, tell me the truth so I can help you."

"You won't tell my wife or anyone will you?" said Bill as his tough exterior started to crumble.

"I am legally bound to keep this confidential." I said bracing myself.

"I don't even want you putting it in my chart," Bill looked straight at me. A shadow of fear crossed his face as he debated telling me the truth.

"Okay, if that is the way you want it, I will just record it as issues discussed."

"I lied when I told you how many pills I'd been taking it's more like twelve a day." Bill shifted his gaze to the floor.

"Bill, I told you that can severely damage your liver!"

"Yeah I heard you, so I made sure some of the pills I took were straight Oxys without Tylenol."

"Where did you get those? Your prescriptions, Dr. Burns and mine, were for oxycodone with Tylenol." I struggled to keep my voice even.

"I have a friend that had some Oxy 10 mg tabs, so I traded."

I pressed my lips together hard. "How long have you been getting these off the street?"

"I don't know, a few months maybe. See Doc, I've been careful not to poison my liver." He looked at me like I should pat him on the back.

"Bill! What are you doing? Now you're dealing with drug pushers on the street. Don't you know that's a felony?"

"I'm just trying to tell the truth. Isn't that what you wanted? If you go and get upset with me why should I be honest with you?"

"Because being honest is the right thing to do. Telling the truth is not something you do for what you get in return. You do it because mutual trust is the basis of healthy relationships," I said trying to understand the scope of Bill's addiction. "What you are telling me still does not add up to the amount of pills you've been prescribed. Don't be throwing out half-truths; that is the same as lying." I sent up a silent prayer for discernment.

"Well, I started buying some from my friend just to help get me through. I knew you wouldn't give me extra, I had nowhere else to turn."

"Go on," I urged, sensing Bill still hadn't told me the whole story.

"Buying Oxys off my friend became expensive, so he suggested something cheaper." At this point Bill began to struggle within himself. "So… so I took his advice and bought a little heroin. But I only smoked it. No needles I would never do that. No one else knows, that's why I don't want you writing this down."

"How much heroin are you using?" I asked becoming alarmed at this turn of events.

"Not much...just two or three bags a day. My friend says

that's a small amount compared to most people. What I am really worried about is if I get drug tested at work I'll lose my job."

"Let's make a few things clear," I said, trying to keep the anger from my voice. "The person you get your drugs from is not your friend. He is a drug dealer, and he just hooked you onto heroin. Second, you are addicted, and it is making you lie and cheat with your family, with me, and above all with yourself. Finally, not only are you flirting with losing your job, but also your family and your life."

"I never thought I would be using heroin," Bill's voice

In the United States, just under 200 people a day die from drug overdose. CDC report August 2018

cracked with sorrow. "Why did God let this happen to me? Why did you give me those Vicodin?"

"I understand your wanting to assign blame somewhere else," I said, determining not to let myself get frustrated. "A lot of people do that as a way to ease their own guilt and shame. But in not taking ownership of this addiction, and being honest with yourself, you make things worse. It will be difficult to get the help you need. "

"The only help I need right now is for you to cover me with oxys so I won't have to use heroin and lose my job. You can do that for a friend, can't you?"

"Shifting responsibility becomes another way to avoid facing the truth, and another excuse to use," I countered.

"So what do you want me to do? Go to an AA meeting and say, 'hello, my name is Bill and I'm addicted to heroin… special thanks to my doctor.'"

My mind spun and I looked away. Bill's words stung. What could I possibly say and not make things worse? I wanted to yell—*You're the one who took more than I ordered!* I felt anger welling up inside… I wanted to grab him by the shirt and shout some sense into him, to defend against his slanderous allegation. I was being sucked into his morass of addiction.

"Lord help!" is all I could think.

"Yeah," Bill went on. "Some help you are. You look down on the drug dealer for giving me drugs, condemn me for not facing the truth, when your own ego hides the fact that you started it."

"My ego!" The words poured from my mind and out my mouth. "You're the one whose pride keeps you locked into denial. You need help, but you keep digging a deeper hole convincing yourself you can handle this when you can't. You need to go to a support group, get a mentor and get serious about getting off these drugs."

Bill shook his head, "I just don't feel comfortable at those AA meetings… besides you said you would help me."

My own words about pride resonated in me—hadn't I fallen into the same trap? I had proudly thought my medical knowledge and abilities could handle Bill's addiction. Condemned by my own words, I realized Bill and I suffered from the same thing, a condition called "I can do this on my own."

"… Doc, did you hear what I just said?" Bill raised his voice to get my attention.

"Sorry, what did you say?"

I said, I am sorry if I offended you. I am just angry and upset over this mess… what I've gotten into… never in a million years did I think I would use heroin. My wife will throw me out of the house if she finds out."

I saw vividly how both Bill and I needed forgiveness. I knew the first step in true humility is to confess my failure before God. Truth was, I didn't want to face my own guilt for enabling Bill's addiction. I paused awkwardly. "Bill, will you forgive me for allowing you to get caught up in addictions?"

Bill looked at me, trying to figure out if I meant what I said.

"Lord," I continued out loud. "I am in need of your forgiveness for enabling Bill, and now seek your wisdom in helping him escape from this horrible pit. I admit I don't know where to begin. Forgive me of my pride that causes me to look down on addictions and on Bill, instead of standing beside him. Our hope is not in our own abilities but in you, and you alone. O Lord, we are in desperate need of you."

Silence filled the room. Then a smile of friendship spread across Bill's face.

"Not exactly the apology I expected to hear..." Bill said, then he started to laugh. "I guess we all have a desperate need. And yes, I forgive you... so where do we go from here?"

~

Most addiction guidelines say you need to sign a pain contract. Then we'll agree on how to schedule the drug taper. The usual regimen people start with is a stable dose of medication that prevents withdrawal. After 30 days we can begin to cut back.

I have had patients who did not want to include God in their dealing with addictions, and I respected their decision. But I cannot disregard my own spiritual need for God's help. To ignore God in life is to walk away from his forgiveness and the Holy Spirit's power for transformation. You settle for trying to prop up the old life on your own effort instead of seeking God's mighty power to make life new.

> *"I pray also that the eyes of your heart may be enlightened in order that you may know the hope to which he has called you, the riches of his glorious inheritance in the saints, and his incomparably great power for us who believe. That power is like the working of his mighty strength, which he exerted in Christ when he raised him from the dead and seated him at his right hand in the heavenly realms." Ephesians 1:18-20*

This doesn't mean that we are transformed without struggling. Asking for God's help isn't about Him doing what we want (i.e., the quick fix), for doing what we want is how we got into this mess. Instead, we are learning to trust Him through all the ups and downs of recovery. We are to seek forgiveness and learn to forgive; to choose his way rather than our way. God is faithful to bring about our restoration as we trust in him, but we are clay in his hands not the other way around.

With great humility King David prayed Psalm 51 spurred by guilt and shame for murdering Uriah to cover up his rape of Bathsheba. It should be our prayer too.

*"Create in me a pure heart, O God,*
*and renew a steadfast spirit within me.*
*Do not cast me from your presence*
*or take your Holy Spirit from me.*
*Restore to me the joy of your salvation*
*and grant me a willing spirit, to sustain me." Psalm 51:10–12*

CHAPTER 4

# Lost and Needing Help

Bill came in a day early for his appointment and demanded to be seen. I only had one more patient before lunch so we put him in an exam room to wait. After finishing the morning schedule, my nurse warned me that Bill seemed upset.

"Bill, you're a day early what gives," I said, sitting down on my stool to face him.

"Yesterday they sent me home from work and I will lose my job unless you can write me a note," Bill twisted his company baseball cap as he talked.

"A note for what? Tell me what's this all about."

"I had an accident with the forklift and they drug tested me on the spot. It came back positive, so I told them you were prescribing pain killers for my back pain. They said if I didn't get a medical verification that I would lose my job. When I got home and told my wife she went ballistic and threatened to kick me out if I didn't get off everything. You have to help me or I'll lose it all."

"I'll give you the note stating I have been prescribing oxycodone, but first I need to test a urine sample for my records."

"But I just got tested can't you use that one?"

"I won't be able to access those records, and I need to record that I am keeping track of you as the drug taper progresses."

"Well, I didn't know you couldn't get the results, so I went just before coming in."

"Then I guess we'll wait here until you can give me a urine specimen."

Bill fidgeted rubbing his index finger with his thumb, looking around for some way to escape.

"Okay," he finally blurted out. "I took some heroin this

morning, because with all this stress I ran out of Oxys, and I couldn't function without something."

The air left the room…I took a deep breath. "I thought your wife kept the pills and only gave you enough for each day?"

"We had a fight and she threatened to throw them out. So I took them back for safe keeping."

I stared at Bill trying to hide my emotions and quickly prayed, What now, Lord? Am I helping or enabling? This is way beyond my ability and wisdom to handle. Jesus, please give me the words to say and the direction to go, for I know you have been given authority over all things, including Bill's addiction.

"Doc, why is God letting this happen to me and my family?" Bill interrupted my prayer. "I've prayed for healing and nothing happens."

"Frankly Bill, I don't know why God doesn't just take away your addiction. But I also don't understand why God allows all sorts of illness. I think it comes down to faith and love. God values our faith in him, and only in tough times does our faith grow. Trusting in his love, even when we don't see it, is somehow good for us in the long run. There is also the issue of choosing to follow him even when it hurts. This life is filled with pain that makes us either commit to him or leave in despair. We must have faith that God loves us, forgives us, and will help us even when we don't see it, or feel it."

"Sometimes I would like him to give me more of the 'feel it' than put me through the 'faith it,'" Bill lamented. "That's the thing about drugs, if I need a little lift I can have it within minutes, but with faith in God I have to wait, and even then I may not get what I want."

"Getting what we want is not always good for us. I think your addiction is a painful example of that."

"That's easy for you to say," Bill responded, "you've never had to go through withdrawal."

"All of us have trouble waiting on God," I admitted. "But I

think one of the biggest problems with drugs is it takes away any ability to wait. Everything has to be right now. You end up trading away any long-term blessing for immediate relief."

The ability to postpone pleasure and to obtain long-term benefits is critical in life, from success at school to showing up for work. Drugs and alcohol rob the mind of that ability. Building it back up is a difficult process that can only begin as one remains sober, fighting the fight.

*"Out of the depths I cry to you, O Lord;*
*O Lord, hear my voice.*
*Let your ears be attentive*
*to my cry for mercy.*
*If you, O Lord, kept a record of sins,*
*O Lord, who could stand?*
*But with you there is forgiveness;*
*therefore you are feared.*
*I wait for the Lord, my soul waits,*
*and in his word I put my hope.*
*My soul waits for the Lord*
*more than watchmen wait for the morning,*
*more than watchmen wait for the morning."*
*Psalm 130:1–6*

"Bill, did you ever wonder why you took a gamble with heroin knowing it could damage your family, cause you to lose your job, and destroy your life?"

"I am not taking heroin regularly. I don't have to have it," Bill protested.

"But you took it this morning. Tell me what would your wife say if she knew you used heroin earlier today?"

"Oh my, she would be furious and kick me out. She already said if I don't get rid of this drug thing soon she will divorce me. She doesn't want our kids growing up watching their dad use drugs."

"Do you agree with her that your kids should not be around someone using drugs?"

"Yes, but..."

"Then why did you take heroin this morning?"

"Just this one time, till I could get in here to see you."

"Bill, drugs have made you a liar and a cheat to your family, to me, but most of all to yourself. I thought we could deal with this, but now I am not sure we can, maybe you need a more structured environment."

"You mean drug rehab."

"Yes, until you really get off these drugs."

"I can't. I told you I can't afford it. I'll lose my home and truck...who is going to feed my family? Please Doc, I promise to do everything you say."

"You're making promises you can't keep."

"What can I say? Give me another chance. If you don't help me I will just have to do it on my own."

"That's the main problem—the underlying deception—you have been thinking all along 'I can do this on my own.' You've resisted participating in a 12-step group. You haven't pushed hard to get a mentor or change your environment. That's why I am recommending going to rehab, for the truth is, you can't do it on your own."

"Okay Doc, maybe I have been fooling myself..."

"There is no maybe about it—when will you let go of your pride and in true humility seek help?"

"I really do want help!" Bill now looked scared. "But my desire for help evaporates with the intensity of withdrawal."

"Now you are starting to be honest with yourself."

"I feel so ashamed, how can God accept me when I don't have the faith or the willpower to stop?"

"It is only when you are humble before the Lord and admit you are powerless over this that you can begin to receive his help. Like the father in Mark 9 asking Jesus to heal his son: '*I believe, help my unbelief.*' Even when your faithfulness is insufficient, you can ask for help."

"Will you help me?" Bill said with tears of fear running down his cheeks. "I don't have the means to go to rehab. Is there any way I can do it here and continue to work? I'll do whatever you say. I really am desperate."

~

The reason drug rehab units can help people is they allow the patient to pull away from life's patterns that trigger use. An example would be traveling down the street where they bought drugs would trigger craving and subsequent use. Drug rehab also provides a very structured environment including group meetings where patients learn about addictions and are encouraged to be transparent with each other. This tight structure keeps the patient engaged in the task at hand and minimizes down time when the thought of using begins to fester. A difficult problem is that many units are not equipped to handle acute withdrawal so they require the incoming patient to be clean. The stay in rehab is voluntary and most have strict rules that if violated get the patient dismissed from the program. There are also rapid detox units, but they only treat physical withdrawal and do not get into psychological or spiritual sides of addiction treatment. Rapid detox centers tend to be expensive and have a poor track record for helping over the long term.

A small church in the Ukraine had the most encouraging program I have seen. It was part of the church's outreach because a majority of the members were former addicts. Everyone worked to support the program either on a nearby farm or in a church-run business. They held each other accountable and went through a 12-step program together. They prayed, ate, and worked together building a cohesive group. Upon completing the program each committed to helping others in their recovery. Building those relationships in the church was integral to the success of each person involved.

Recovery from drugs is successful when old drug related patterns are broken off and new relationships are formed with people who will hold each other accountable. This changing of drug related patterns is also true for the family, old codependent behavior has to be changed or it will pull the person back into using.

CHAPTER 5

# The Seven Lies of Addictions

Four weeks later, Bill had just finished a month on a stabilizing dose of Oxycodone. This would begin the start of going to a lower dose. His vacation had come and gone with various reasons put forth as to why he couldn't completely taper off. The primary reason being that just getting down to a stabilized dose of seventy milligrams a day involved a lot of effort. I had his wife, Laura, controlling the pills and doled them out one day at a time.

"Okay Bill, we need a urine drug screen for this visit," I said on walking into the exam room.

"I didn't know you were going to want a urine sample today. I just went before coming in," Bill protested.

"Then drink some water," I shrugged. "And have a seat in the waiting room until you're ready."

"Doc, can I come back and give you a specimen tomorrow? I have to pick up my kids at day care."

"Bill you signed a contract stating you would come to each visit prepared to give a urine sample and if not, you wouldn't get a prescription." Red flags went up in my mind that things were not going well.

"I forgot," whined Bill. "Give me a break just this once. I'll come prepared to give you urine on all my future visits…I promise."

"Bill you already agreed to do that by signing the contract. I can't give you a prescription without checking your urine."

"You're treating me like some back-alley doper. We've known each other for years, isn't that worth something? You're supposed to be helping me not make it tougher." Bill's voice became loud. "If you don't give me a prescription, you'll be forcing me to get stuff off the street. You want that hanging over your head?"

"Bill, you're trying to manipulate me and suggests you're hiding something."

"Okay Doc, you tell me what to do," Bill said with annoyance. "I have to pick up the kids or we get charged a huge amount for each minute I am late to daycare. I can't go through withdrawal when I'm the only one at home to watch my kids. There is no good alternative if you don't give me a prescription."

I felt trapped, but I figured if Bill was hiding something it would eventually come out. So I caved and gave him a prescription for six Oxys per day for one week.

"Hey," Bill complained. "You gave me only forty-two, that's not enough for two weeks at seven a day."

"One week at six a day as per our taper agreement. In one week, come in to give me a urine specimen and I'll give you another prescription. You signed the plan that after one month of seven a day we would go to six a day," I reminded him.

"Yeah, but most of the month I struggled to just get down to seven pills a day. I am still not used to this level. Cut me some slack for one more week at seven a day to catch my breath," countered Bill.

"I never said this would be pain-free. The lower level will be uncomfortable for a few days but then you will readjust."

"Easy for you to say," Bill shot back, "but you're not the one going through this. I just need a few good days to get myself together again."

"You think the drug makes your day good, but that's the addiction talking. Life is not about feeling good; it's about the goodness found in family and friends. Real joy is not in what Oxycodone can give you," I said. "It's in giving joy to those around you. Think of your family."

"Doc, I am thinking of my family—when I am going through withdrawal, I am no joy to be around."

"Have you been going to AA meetings?" I said trying to decide how much to believe Bill. "What about a mentor to help you over these rough patches?"

"Nah, I haven't really had a chance to connect with a mentor. I am either working or taking care of kids, so I haven't made many meetings; besides, I'm not really like any of them."

"You need to have an accountability group—people to help you in the same way you need to help them."

"My wife and kids are all the help I need," said Bill.

"But you can manipulate them too easily, and they will have difficulty seeing through the lies you tell yourself. I must say your reluctance joining others in the struggle to stay sober is a sign you still don't see the depth of your desperate situation."

"Don't worry, Doc, I do know..." Bill sat there looking at the prescription. "My wife will keep me accountable."

"You don't understand. She is your wife and often family are codependent. She probably needs others to point out where she is enabling you. Maybe I should talk with her."

"Why?"

"Just to make sure she understands. I need your permission of course."

"Well, I'll think about it, but I just don't see how I can do all this stuff and earn a living. Now you are throwing in another office visit on top of everything plus having my wife come in. This is getting way too complicated and expensive...Why are you making this so hard?"

My stomach went into a knot with his words. "Bill, I think you're hiding from the truth..."

"I've got to get going," said Bill. "I can't stay and argue, so I guess I'll have to come back in a week." Taking the prescription he shot out the door.

The next week, Bill came in and gave us a urine specimen that showed positive for oxycodone and a faint positive for other opiates.

"Bill, have you taken anything besides my prescription for

oxycodone?" I asked trying to be careful not to sound accusatory.

"I'm getting sick and tired of everyone calling me a liar, my dad, my wife, now you," growled Bill. "What do I have to do to get some respect? Everyone treats me like some skid row addict."

The lying and misdirection with addictions is a constant problem, and the last person to recognize it is the one using. Rationalization is the term commonly used to dress up the lies making them seem not quite so vile, yet whatever you call them, the outcome is the same—hiding from the truth. I have listed seven lies I've encountered over the years (though I realize there are many more):

- At least I am not like…
- I can control this, I just need a little more time.
- If I can just have some now, then I'll have strength to tackle the problem.
- I need this to function and think normally.
- This isn't my fault, so why should I be the one to suffer? (It is just not fair).
- I can't forgive myself / I can't forgive them.
- I am hopeless, what is the use. I am bent and can't be fixed.

"Trust is easily lost and takes a long time to build up," I said.

"So what am I to do in the meantime?" Bill looked annoyed.

"Do what's right, be merciful, and walk in humility before God," I responded.

Bill just sat there not speaking.

"Okay so tell me," I finally said. "Did you take anything besides what I prescribed? Be honest, or I'll send the urine into a lab and they'll tell me."

"Not really," said Bill.

"What do you mean not really?"

"I… I only got morphine off the street to replace the Oxys Laura took from me. That's why I end up short sometimes. She has a problem too."

My mind reeled with this new twist to Bill's addiction. I didn't know what to believe.

"What are you thinking? You can't let someone else use your prescription. That's a felony!" I exclaimed. "I want to talk with Laura right now. I need to clear this up."

"I don't want Laura to know I told you," Bill said emphatically. "We are having enough problems; you talking to her will just make things worse between us."

"I think things are pretty bad right now, but I can't talk to her without your permission."

My mind raced trying to get a handle on what to do next. Part of me didn't believe Bill and felt he might be using this accusation to hide continued street drug use. Also, I knew Laura from church and she didn't seem to fit with Bill's accusation.

Bill went on, "Well, for now, I want to handle it. I'll just keep my own prescription locked up and away from her."

"Bill, I need to talk to Laura or I won't give you further prescriptions for oxycodone."

"Hey, what gives? I try to be honest about things, and now you want to cut me off!" Bill complained.

"I didn't say I would cut you off, but I can't help you if I only know parts of the story. I need to communicate freely to all the people involved in your addiction—that includes Laura."

"Well, I've told you the whole story," Bill seemed irritated. "What else do you need to know, my shoe size?"

"Cut out the sarcasm Bill, I've trusted your claims that you have told me the whole story before, and I only find myself getting blindsided by new revelations."

"Okay, have it your way," Bill snapped. "But at least give me a chance to talk with Laura first then you can talk with her."

"I will give you one week's supply of oxycodone. If by next visit Laura hasn't called me, then we're done."

"You're really making it hard on me," Bill grumbled as he left with his prescription.

Returning to my office after Bill left I did not know what to think. I realized with Bill I could not discern the truth from the lies because he sincerely believed them himself. As for Laura, I looked forward to talking with her and getting a different perspective. But what if she really was addicted too?

~

The truth is that anyone can become addicted, just like we all struggle with pride and lying. Pride is a cunning deceiver and hides the truth about ourselves. Like it did for the Pharisee:

*"To some who were confident of their own righteousness and looked down on everybody else, Jesus told this parable: 'Two men went up to the temple to pray, one a Pharisee and the other a tax collector. The Pharisee stood up and prayed about himself: 'God, I thank you that I am not like other men—robbers, evildoers, adulterers—or even like this tax collector. I fast twice a week and give a tenth of all I get.'*
*But the tax collector stood at a distance. He would not even look up to heaven, but beat his breast and said, 'God, have mercy on me, a sinner.'*
*I tell you that this man, rather than the other, went home justified before God. For everyone who exalts himself will be humbled, and he who humbles himself will be exalted." Luke 18:9-14 NIV*

Everyone who tells a lie after a while begins to believe the lie…

*"They exchanged the truth of God for a lie, and worshiped and*

*served created things rather than the Creator—who is forever praised. Amen." Romans 1:25 NIV*

...and everyone who believes a lie becomes its slave.

*"I tell you the truth, everyone who sins is a slave to sin." –Jesus, John 8:34 NIV*

Only the truth can set you free.

*"Jesus said, 'If you hold to my teaching, you are really my disciples. Then you will know the truth, and the truth will set you free.'" John 8:31-32 NIV*

Celebrate Recovery's first principle is based on Matthew 5:3 (a truth for all of us). "Realize I'm not God; I admit that I am powerless to control my tendency to do the wrong thing and that my life is unmanageable. *'Happy are those who know that they are spiritually poor.'*" Acknowledging the poorness of our spiritual state leads to humbly asking for God's help.

To counter the lies that drugs and alcohol push upon those under their spell, the person must continually be reminded of the truth. That is part of the purpose of joining an accountability group. This is not about reciting platitudes, but digging into the real truth that can expose the lies and lead to freedom.

A review of God's truth for our lies:

The lie: "At least I am not like..."

*"When pride comes, then comes disgrace, but with humility comes wisdom." Proverbs 11:2 NIV*

The lie: "I can control this, I just need a little more time."

*"He who trusts in his own heart is a fool, but whoever walks wisely will be delivered." Proverbs 28:26 NKJV*

The lie: "If I can just have some now, then I'll have strength to tackle the problem. I need this to function and think normally."

*"Some trust in chariots and some in horses, but we trust in the name of the LORD our God." Psalm 20:7 NIV*

The lie: "This isn't my fault, so why should I be the one to suffer? (It is just not fair)."

*"In this world you will have trouble. But take heart! I have overcome the world." - Jesus, John 16:33 NIV*

The lie: "I can't forgive myself / I can't forgive them."

*"Yet the LORD longs to be gracious to you; He rises to show you compassion." Isaiah 30:18 NIV*

The lie: "I am hopeless, what is the use. I am bent and can't be fixed."

*"A bruised reed He will not break, a smoldering wick He will not snuff out, till He leads justice to victory." Matthew 12:20 NIV*

The truth: "God is on your side. He loves you dearly."

CHAPTER 6

# The Three Sides of Addiction

Bill missed his next appointment. I immediately called his home to find out why. Laura answered.

"This is Doctor Hufman. Is Bill home?"

"Doctor Hufman, I'm worried something has happened. Bill didn't come home from work last night. He has been pretty agitated the last two days... I hope he has not done anything stupid." Laura's voice shook with worry.

She didn't have to say it but both of us were worried he had overdosed.

"Do you know where he might be, or any places he would go?" I asked.

"The only place I can think of is a spot along Kootenai River where he and his dad went fishing, just the other side of milepost 36. But I can't leave because of the kids, and my car is in the shop."

"I'll go," I said. There were no more patients on the schedule and I knew I wouldn't be able to stop worrying.

"Oh, doctor, thank you. He has a black Ford pickup with a 'Get high with Jesus' bumper sticker." She sighed. "I can't believe he put that sticker on his pickup, but I think it's his way of dealing with his shame. You have to find him before he does something stupid."

I tried to reassure her, but I had no idea what I might find. Just after marker 36, I spotted Bill's truck tucked off the road with the bumper sticker Laura had described. "Lord Jesus, we need your help now. Please let me find Bill alive."

Not wanting to announce my presence I parked further down the road and walked back through the woods on a fisherman's trail. There next to the river, Bill crouched over a camp fire feeding it sticks, behind him he had erected a tent.

I cleared my throat to let him know I was near. "Bill, what are you doing here? You missed our appointment and your family has been worried."

Bill stood in shock at seeing me. Suddenly from the tent a woman emerged and stood beside Bill.

Words stumbled from Bill's mouth. "Doc! How... Ah, what are you doing here... This is my friend, Connie... she is like a sister... I had to get away and get myself together... I do much better out here by the river."

"What about your medication? You missed your appointment."

"Oh, I'm okay, I am going to do a fast taper out here and be done with it. Connie is going to help me... with nowhere to go it will be a lot easier."

"But what about your family?" I asked. "You didn't tell them anything, you just disappeared. They are worried sick."

"I had to get away to get this done," said Bill. "It was just too hard to do it with them around; I needed some space. Tell them I am okay and will get in touch when this is over. Believe me, they are better off without me around right now."

"I don't agree. You'll need their support to get through this."

"Doc, I know what I am doing, besides Connie is here, she'll keep me on course." Bill said putting his arm on Connie's shoulder.

"That's just the point. I don't think this way honors God. Maybe you both need help." I said looking at Connie, who seemed to be a little lethargic and wobbly.

"You're wrong, Doc, but thanks for stopping by to check on me, this way will be easier, you'll see." Bill turned his back toward me and began to add sticks to the fire and Connie ducked back into the tent.

"Bill, there is no easy way except the wrong way," I said. But Bill was done. He ignored me and would not listen anymore. I stood there a few awkward minutes and finally turned and left.

Upon returning home, I called Laura to let her know I had

talked with Bill. “He’s safe. He decided it would be easier to rapid taper off drugs in the woods and be done with withdrawal.” I did not say anything about Connie.

“I don’t know, Doc. I called Bill’s boss at the mill to see if they knew where he might be; they said he had been absent from work for three days and no longer has a job. Then I checked for our grocery money and it’s all gone.”

“You think Bill took it?” I asked already knowing the answer.

“I know he did because he has done it before to buy drugs,” Laura began to cry.

“How are you going to feed the kids?” I asked.

“My parents will help us out. They won’t let their grandchildren starve.”

“Laura, there is something else I have to ask you.” I took a deep breath. “Have you used any of Bill’s oxycodone?”

“What?” Laura gasped. “What has Bill been saying about me?” Her voice tinged with anger and disbelief.

“I can’t talk to you about my conversations with Bill,” I said. “But I must know the truth to be able to help both of you.”

“He gave me some of his oxycodone when I complained of a headache. I took one but didn’t like how it made me feel. Then he showed me how he snorts it, and urged me to try it that way. I got pretty upset and threatened to flush the pills down the toilet. I would have, but then he said you had told him to take them this way. Did you tell him that? With Bill I don’t know what to believe anymore.”

“Of course not!” I gasped in disbelief. “I would never prescribe narcotics to be snorted. Bill has been telling lies to manipulate us. The scope and depth of his addiction is greater than I realized. In the future, I will communicate with you personally by phone; we are not going to be able to trust anything Bill says. Do you have any drugs about the house now?”

“No, I am sure Bill took all of that with him.”

“Double check and if you find any pain meds or anything

that you don't know what it is, get rid of it."

"Frankly, Doctor Hufman, I'm getting sick and tired of his lies and being played the fool. Bill may think this is an easy way, but he sure is making it hard on everyone else. I have prayed and prayed for Bill, but he just doesn't seem to care. I don't know how much more I can take."

After the phone call with Laura I slumped down in the chair. Lord, what is going on? Help Laura and her family… Wake up Bill to what he is doing. Why don't you just slap Bill upside the head and fix it? I began to wonder how many times Bill's family had prayed pleading to God for help only to have things fall apart.

*"Consider it pure joy, my brothers, whenever you face trials of many kinds, because you know that the testing of your faith develops perseverance. Perseverance must finish its work so that you may be mature and complete, not lacking anything." James 1:2-4 NIV*

This verse from James appears to be cruel on the surface, but it speaks to an essential part of life that is critical in overcoming addictions--perseverance. God wants to develop this in our lives and it can only be done trusting Him in the face of adversity.

*"That is why we never give up. Though our bodies are dying, our spirits are being renewed every day. For our present troubles are small and won't last very long. Yet they produce for us a glory that vastly outweighs them and will last forever! So we don't look at the troubles we can see now; rather, we fix our gaze on things that cannot be seen. For the things we see now will soon be gone, but the things we cannot see will last forever." 2 Corinthians 4:16-18 NIV*

Drugs destroy our perseverance, getting us to rely on a quick fix of chemical pleasure that is temporary and enslaving. On the flip side God uses trials to develop perseverance and reliance upon Him. It is a spiritual tug-of-war.

> *"Not only so, but we also rejoice in our sufferings, because we know that suffering produces perseverance; perseverance, character; and character, hope. And hope does not disappoint us, because God has poured out his love into our hearts by the Holy Spirit, whom he has given us." Romans 5:3-5 NIV*

~

A few weeks later Bill's parents John and Martha called.

"Doctor Hufman, we wanted to let you know we have heard from Bill. He is on the streets in Spokane and wants us to wire him some money. We are pretty torn up over the mess he has made of his life and family. Laura is divorcing him, says she can't take it anymore, and that she doesn't want the kids seeing him in a drug stupor. We don't blame her. But he is still our son. What should we do?"

"I am afraid if you send him money it will just go to buying more drugs," I said. "If you want to go to Spokane and try to get him into drug treatment, that would be positive."

"We have tried to help in the past," Bill's mother said, "but things just seem to get worse. We barely make it on John's pension from the mill and we can't afford much in the way of treatment. Though we'd do almost anything, even re-mortgage the house if we knew it would help. We just don't know what is the right thing to do."

Everyone in Bill's family felt like they were on a roller coaster, their hopes way up when Bill was filled with contrition and entered rehab, only to have them dashed when he would relapse after getting out. The divorce hit Bill hard; unfortunately it became another excuse to take drugs. He even tried to get Laura to relent by threatening to overdose if she didn't give him another chance. Laura told me that threat was exactly why she had to get out—emotionally she could not take anymore. There were weeks when the family heard nothing, then would come a barrage of phone calls from Bill pleading for money couched in promises of getting help. Then came a call from the Spokane Police. Bill had been found unconscious in a stolen vehicle. He was put in jail after a visit to the ER for the overdose drug Narcan. Bail had been set at $10,000, and the police were calling to see if anyone wanted to post bail.

Bill's parents went to visit, but refused to post bail.

"You can't leave me in here. I'm sick and need help," Bill pleaded through the glass.

"We want you to know we love you, but we don't have the money for bail, nor do we know how to keep you from using drugs."

"I'm going to die in here! I'm your son. You have to do something."

"We'll visit with you as much as we are able, and we will be praying for you."

"Times up," said the guard. "You have to return to your cell."

Back in his cell, Bill broke down in the torment of his life, how he had lost everything, and now in jail he had nothing but the shakes and retching of addiction.

"God, why? How could you let this happen? If you exist, help me." Bill's whole body shook, and he curled in a ball. Intermittently, he heaved over the toilet then the shakes would start up again. "Lord, take my life. I'd rather die than this," he sobbed. His thoughts stuck on dying… losing his life… a worthless miserable life. A Bible verse popped into his mind: *For whoever wants to save his life will lose it, but whoever loses his life for me will save it.* In the midst of his agony Bill saw clearly—he desperately wanted to lose his life.

"Jesus, take my life!" Bill cried out. He retched so hard his stomach cramped, pulling him to his knees, he held the toilet bowl to keep from falling into it. "Jesus, take me, I beg YOU!"

More words found their way into Bill's tortured mind: *It is not the healthy who need a doctor, but the sick. I have not come to call the righteous, but sinners to repentance.*

"I am so sick," Bill said as he looked at his reflection in the toilet bowl. "Help me, Jesus! I need you."

Bill continued with the shakes and vomiting for another two days, but there was one difference—he let his life go, and put his hope in God.

About a year after Bill got out of jail, we met for breakfast. He had been clean since his release and I wanted to know what had happened.

Bill began, "Being locked in jail going through withdrawal had to be the worst days of my life, but also the most blessed, for there in that cell I had to face the truth. I realized my whole life I had been play-acting about asking God for forgiveness-- never really wanting to change. But when the shame is so great you would rather die than go on living, that's where you have to decide whom you are going to follow. I had to give up the right to end my life and let Jesus be in charge. I literally had to lose my life to find it. Denying my own desires and feelings, I had to pick up that cross and follow Him. I never understood the shame of the cross of Christ until now… it is my shame on that cross, but He bares it for me. I just have to walk with Him, leaning on Him, trusting in Him."

"So, God healed you there in prison?" I asked.

"Yes… and no. Jesus gave me new life in him, but I still went through a tough physical withdrawal. It lasted four days, and I never want to do that again. After withdrawal, I had to work through a lot of junk my mind believed."

"But God did heal you?" I pressed.

Bill sat there a moment thinking, then looked me in the eye. "I still get these voices bringing up all my failures, accusing me of being a terrible father, telling me I am a worthless addict, that my family would be better off without me. All of it trying to get me to take a little pill to feel right again. So in that sense I am not healed. I have to go to meetings and talk with my mentor and keep working through the steps of recovery. On a daily basis I have to remind myself of God's grace and be very careful not to fall into the trap of pride—the 'I can take it from here' type thing. On the other hand, I know that there is now no condemnation for me in Christ Jesus… so yes, I am healed."

"Wow, that's great," I said at a loss for words. "I'm glad to hear you're keeping close with your support group."

I started to get up from the table to leave when Bill grabbed my arm.

"I need to say one more thing about God's healing," Bill said causing me to sit down again. "Even though there are times I don't feel healed, I have to hold on to the fact that Jesus loves me, and I am forgiven. God is teaching me to wait. Drugs' allure is that you can have it all now. Like you said, they destroy any ability to wait. Not being able to wait destroyed my marriage, hurt my family and left me with nothing. Now, Jesus is teaching me to wait on Him. His grace covers all my mistakes in the past and every day until He takes me home. Each day I am learning to walk by faith and not by feelings. It is the hardest thing I have ever done, yet I know it is not by my hard work that I will make it, but by the love and power of God. Through all this I cling to the words—nothing can separate me from His love. That is the healing Jesus has done for me. It is built upon his strength not mine, and I would have it no other way. I have been trying to live by Psalm 27: *'Teach me your way, O LORD, and lead me in a level path…I believe I shall see the goodness of the LORD in the land of the living. Wait for the LORD; be strong and let your heart take courage; wait for the LORD!'*" Bill lowered his eyes and after a long pause added, "I am trying to learn how to wait and it is hard. There is no easy way except waiting and trusting in God."

I have thought a lot about Bill since that last meeting and continue to pray for him. But more importantly, I have come to see how what he said to me is true for all of us. Now my prayers always end with: "Thank you, Jesus. I wait for You."

Three aspects of dealing with addictions need to be addressed:

1. Physical: The effect of the particular drugs on various organs of the body result in withdrawal symptoms when the drug is stopped. On the opposite end, when too much drug is taken, it can lead to respiratory depression and death. Immediate treatment with Narcan is required.

2. Psychological: This can be seen in the behavioral changes that occur in addictions. Some more common are: A continued craving for drugs long after physical withdrawal has subsided. A reduced capability to say no to drugs. The alteration of brain neural chemicals making the brain more susceptible to depression, anxiety, and paranoia._The brain loses its ability to choose, being rewired by the addiction into compulsive behavior. The time of exposure for this to happen varies depending on the substance, the genetics of the person, and age (younger brains exhibit more plasticity and therefore are more vulnerable).

3. Spiritual/heart: This is where pride, humility, guilt, shame, anger, blame, lying, forgiveness, and trust reside. I am sure the list is longer but what is important is that the spiritual side of addictions cannot be ignored or glossed over lest we fail to understand our greatest need. It reminds me of the verse in Zechariah that expresses our need for addressing the spiritual in addictions.

*"'Not by might nor by power, but by my Spirit,' says the Lord Almighty." Zachariah 4:6 NIV*

These three areas of need extend beyond the person who is addicted. Family and friends need God's help to hang in there during the tough times, and to discern when they are getting caught up in the addiction as enablers. There is a weariness that comes when you try to help someone with addictions; you swing between wanting to knock some sense into them, or wanting to give up and walk away. As one parent confided in me, "I am so ashamed, for there are times I wish he would just overdose and put an end to this misery." Waking up to our desperate need for God's help is the first step to right living, and the second step is to do it daily.

*"If anyone would come after me, he must deny himself and take up his cross daily and follow me. For whoever wants to save his life will lose it, but whoever loses his life for me will save it." Luke 9:23-24 NIV*

SECTION 2

# Hope for the Hopeless

For many who live in the trenches of this horrible war with drugs and alcohol, the first word to hold onto is hope. Not "I hope I get lucky," or "I hope it turns out okay," but real hope of a life free from this terrible curse. We have all heard marvelous stories of people waking up one day and deciding they have had enough and never looking back. No doubt some have thrown off addictions by sheer force of self-determination, but for most, having this huge force of will is beyond their capability. What we all are looking for is a story of hope for the weakest among us—to hear there is hope for the poor soul who has no soul left. A hope that can make up for a squandered life, hope of rescue when the Grim Reaper has all but closed the deal. Hope that doesn't run out when we fall for the umpteenth time and we give up on ourselves. That kind of powerful hope is what we need to break the control of this dark power.

*"One of the criminals who hung there hurled insults at him: 'Aren't you the Christ? Save yourself and us!' But the other criminal rebuked him. 'Don't you fear God,' he said, 'since you are under the same sentence? We are punished justly, for we are getting what our deeds deserve. But this man has done nothing wrong.' Then he said, 'Jesus, remember me when you come into your kingdom.' Jesus answered him, 'I tell you the truth, today you will be with me in paradise.'" Luke 23:39-43*

Truly hope for the hopeless.

CHAPTER 7

# Give Me Something

Before entering the exam room of my next patient, I looked through his chart and read the nurse's note: 50-year-old male needs medication, may have drug addiction problem. Upon opening the door, I encountered a disheveled old man, slumped into the chair like a pile of rags. "There must be some mistake," I thought.

He looked up at me his eyes showed fear mixed with apprehension.

"Hello, Lester. I am Dr. Hufman. How can I help you?" I asked, extending my hand, but he sat there. His clothes were unkempt and frayed at the edges reeking of tobacco. He had a gray unkempt beard and a wrinkled leathery face. His yellow teeth were a witness of a tough life with half of them gone, and those left seemed hardly worth keeping. He had not an ounce of cheer in his body.

"I need you to give me something for my nerves, I…I can't live like this," he said, his eyes darting about the room searching as if someone were after him.

Knowing why he had come in, I asked, "And what 'something' are you seeking with this visit?"

"Don't jerk me around, Doc; I know your nurse told you about me, the meds I need. I'm talking about Percs, White Stuff, or better yet—give me methadone."

"Whoa. Slow down there. This isn't the town soda fountain."

"Listen, Doc. If you don't give me methadone or somethin' I'll go back on the streets to get junk. If I do that, the police will try to send me back to jail and I'd rather die than go back there."

"Well, there are consequences to your actions," I said.

"Maybe you should clean up if you don't want to return to prison."

"Doc, you don't know nothing. I am a junk-head—I'd rather have the cops shoot me dead than lock me up. You want a police killin' hanging over your head? So you better give me something, or else…"

"Oh my," I said, a little shocked at his threat. "You're going too fast for me to keep up. Please, tell me how you came to such a desperate condition."

> Addiction definition:
>
> 1. The condition of being addicted to a particular substance, thing, or activity.
>
> 2. Compulsive need for and use of a habit-forming substance (such as heroin, nicotine, or alcohol) characterized by tolerance to the substance, and by well-defined physiological symptoms upon withdrawal.
>
> 3. Persistent use of a substance known by the user to be harmful.

"I don't think you want to know about that," Lester replied slumping back in the chair. "Besides, I am not sure I want to go into it. So, just gimme the stuff."

"Well, I can't help you unless I get a full history. If you won't cooperate then save us both the time…"

"Okay, you asked for it," he said with growing despair. "I have been using since I was sixteen. It started with marijuana and booze, but by the time I hit twenty I had tried cocaine, meth, and all sorts of other junk. But, once I shot up with

> It is estimated that 80-90% of addictions start in adolescent and young adult years. Usually with heavy recreational drug use (marijuana, alcohol, and nicotine).

smack—that was the beginning of the end."

"Why did you ever start?"

A look of disgust and horror came over him, "I got started when my uncle introduced me to marijuana; he got me high on weekends at his place. My dad drank a lot and beat me terrible. So, I moved in with my uncle. That's when we started tokin' every night. Then he told me how I could get even higher by combining it with alcohol. We did that and I usually passed out. One time I woke up with my pants off, laying in bed. My uncle told me he had tried to get me undressed for bed but gave up halfway. I knew something wasn't right but felt too ashamed to confront him. I smoked weed and drank almost every night. Some nights, I'd get real sick, so my uncle gave me pills to get high. That's when he demanded I help pay for it by selling myself. I felt so ashamed of what he had me do that I had to take the pills to forget. When my habit became too expensive, my uncle started givin' me smack. A few years later, my uncle died of an overdose. When the paramedics left with my uncle's body, I got busted for possession, and in searching the house the cops found all kinds of terrible pictures of..." Lester paused as if the next words were too awful to utter.

"Yes, go on," I said.

"My uncle made me do all sorts of terrible things...things I am too ashamed to speak about...okay, are you satisfied now? Do you know what they do to people like me in jail? I got beat and abused so much I have constant pain. When I got out of jail they made me register with the police as a sex offender, the schools know, the community knows...No one wants to be around me. My life is a living hell and there is no way out. Who wants me? I don't even want me. So you gotta give me some pills to quiet the pain, or I'll get in some gun battle with police and end this misery."

My mind reeled. I thought of the agony and shame he must endure. Lord, how do I respond to this man's torment?

"I'm sorry to hear you had such a horrendous life," I said.

"But I need to inform you I can only prescribe methadone for a tapering program. I am not licensed to run a methadone maintenance clinic."

> Methadone maintenance clinics have to be approved and licensed by the FDA. This requires a lot of work to obtain and maintain this designation.

"So you won't help me?"

"No, that's not what I'm saying. I will help you to get off of drugs, but not for drug maintenance. That needs to be understood from the beginning or we will spend our time butting heads—this is not a maintenance program. We will work together to taper you off narcotics however long that takes."

"What about my pain?" he snapped.

"We'll work on other non-narcotic ways to deal with it." I said trying to be reassuring.

"What kind of help is that? My life is too messed up! I have no future. I need something to ease all this now…I don't need no stinking program."

"Sorry, I can't do it any other way. If you want maintenance the nearest methadone clinic is in Spokane."

"How is that going to help? I can't travel that far— you might as well take me out and shoot me. All this talk is getting me upset and you don't want to be around when I get mad," Lester threatened. He then reached behind his waist and pulled out a Bowie knife. "This is what I use for protection on the street."

Lord, what now? I silently prayed.

"Tell me, Lester. What is your hope?" The words just popped out of my mouth.

"Hope? I have no hope except that you give me what I need," growled Lester.

"Maybe that's part of the problem," the words kept tumbling out. "You need hope in something bigger than your addiction, a hope that can cover your past and give you new life."

"Yeah, and while you're at it how about wings so I can fly," said Lester with a snort. He then sheathed the knife and put it away.

"Lester, I'm serious," I said glad to see the knife put away. "More is at stake than procuring methadone and staying out of jail. There is a spiritual part of this that you need to consider. Here's a script with Bible verses about men, just like you with no hope. Please read it, then I want you to go see my friend Dave. He is a leader for the local AA meeting. You need to get into an accountability group to hear others recount their struggles, and how they found help."

"What, so we can all cry on each other's shoulders?" mocked Lester.

"Oh, come on. You're just making excuses to not go. When what you need is to hear stories of hope."

"Okay, I'll meet with Dave and go to one meeting, if that's what it takes to get a prescription from you."

"Lester, I will help you regardless of whether you go to meetings or read the Bible story I gave you, but you know as well as I that your problems run deeper than your addiction."

"Naw, it's okay. I would rather make it a trade for your help, at least that way I am doing something."

"It's a deal," I said, writing out a prescription for methadone. "I am willing to take it one week at a time. See you in seven days. Guard those pills because I won't make up for any shortfalls. And one other thing, please don't bring your knife in here."

"And where do you propose I put it, there are no lock boxes on the street?" said Lester. "Besides it's my protection."

"Well, it doesn't make me feel safe," I protested.

Lester grumped as he left.

*Should I kick him out if he shows up again with the knife?* I wondered. It made me apprehensive about future visits. As I watched him go down the hall I felt the Holy Spirit nudge me, "Where is your hope?"

CHAPTER 8

# Hope Overflowing

A week later, Lester returned to my office, and immediately I noticed a difference. Walking into his presence no longer felt toxic to life. He looked at me and smiled; his tooth-gapped grin reminded me of a happy Halloween pumpkin.

"You'll be happy to know I've been to three meetings of AA, and I met four times with Dave." Lester said with pride. "He agreed to be my mentor."

"Good for you..." I said, amazed at the startling change in Lester's demeanor.

"Dave even helped me read the Bible verses you gave me."

It was then I realized Lester couldn't read, but had been too ashamed to admit it.

"We've been talking about the story of how Jesus had the power to save that totally out-of-control madman runnin' around in that graveyard. No one could help him, but Jesus did. That's just like me. Dave also read me the story of the thief dying on the cross next to Jesus. If Jesus could do that for those two men, I figure he can do something with my worthless life. So I asked Him into my life."

I stood there speechless.

"You know, Doc, I am not afraid of life anymore. I have hope for tomorrow. I don't know how, but Jesus is in charge, and I trust him to bring me through all this to be with him. But best of all, I am forgiven. I have done some terrible things and hurt a lot of people, yet somehow I know God will take care of it. I am also working on forgiving my uncle and my parents; you know hate can be a heavy weight to carry."

"That's...incredible! Wonderful," I sputtered, trying to hide my shock.

"And I'm not afraid of what the future holds, so I don't need to carry the knife anymore," Lester smiled. "Dave has it for safe keeping."

"I'm so glad to hear that," I said, sending up a silent prayer of thanks.

"I tried to stop cold turkey, but the withdrawal became too severe. Dave told me not to worry, that it is okay if I am still addicted. I just need to trust Jesus will save me like he did those other men. So I would like to try a slow taper." Lester looked at me; his face shining like a child asking to go out and play.

"That's great," I said. "We can begin by dropping a quarter tablet every other day. Methadone is long-acting so you will not notice any change for about a week. I will see you then and assess how you are doing."

I gave him a prescription for just one week, along with instructions. We agreed that Dave would keep his pills to avoid any mix up and he would attend AA meetings daily.

"Funny thing about all this," said Lester. "I am truly excited to begin."

I would like to say Lester had smooth sailing and his addiction miraculously disappeared, but he struggled and fell back repeatedly. Fortunately, Dave would not let Lester fall too far. He helped Lester forgive himself and got him back into meetings to work on his recovery. On one notable occasion, Lester found a little package of heroin in a parking lot near his apartment. On his next visit with me he reported what happened:

"When I picked it up I knew, I should have tossed it in the trash," said Lester with a shrug. "But I made up some silly excuse that some kid might find it and OD, so I took it home to flush it down the toilet. When I got home I hesitated and decided to flush it later. Only later, I couldn't get it out of my mind. I thought of calling Dave, but then felt I should be strong enough to handle this. That night I couldn't go to sleep, it kept bugging me, so I took a little bit and snorted it."

"How much have you been using?" I asked, my disappointment showing.

"Well, that's the funny thing," Lester said, shaking his head in disbelief. "When I started to sniff it, I began coughing and couldn't stop. It got so bad I coughed up some blood. Seeing blood really scared me and I flushed the heroin down the toilet. Dave and I think it was God holding onto me."

"Are you still coughing?" I asked.

"Yeah, a little."

"Is there blood in it?"

"I don't know I am afraid to look." Lester said.

"Just to be cautious, let's get a chest x-ray to make sure you're not getting a pneumonia or something."

"Oh Doc, it's just God's way of warning me and pulling me back to Himself." Lester dismissed my concern.

"I believe you, Lester. But, to be safe, I think we should still get a chest x-ray."

The chest x-ray revealed a large mass in his right lung. I sent him off to see an oncologist, who did a thorough work up and diagnosed inoperable lung cancer widely metastatic; palliative care the only option. I had been maintaining Lester's methadone during the work up and now it would be pointless to taper him off. Instead I saw him every other week to make sure he remained comfortable, and on a stable dose.

A short time later during an office visit, Lester reflected on life. "Funny thing about all this, my whole life I have been scared of dying. Foolishly, I sought help in all the wrong places. Relying on things that were actually killing me and robbing me of life. But now that I have terminal cancer, I've found life in dying, like that thief on the cross next to Jesus. My hope in Jesus covers everything with life, even my approaching death. I'm not afraid anymore with Jesus. I am actually looking forward to meeting Him, because I know He has forgiven my horrible past and set me free. Blessed are the poor in spirit, like me, for with Jesus, they receive the kingdom of heaven."

Lester taught me a lot about life, and he had an impact on the entire office. One incident involved his disheveled appearance. To look at him you would label Lester the epitome of a down and out drug addict. A moniker that bothered him.

"Ya know when people see me as worthless it makes it hard not to think of myself the same way," said Lester one day during his office visit. "It becomes one more thing I have to fight through. I know that God has forgiven me and calls me His child. But when I am treated as dirt I begin to believe it and say what's the use."

"You have to admit that years of a hard life using drugs has taken its toll." I said without thinking.

"Thanks a lot, whose side are you on?"

"I'm sorry, that came out wrong." I apologized.

"People think they are so highfalutin, that they could never be caught by addictions but they're no different from me. Most people start using drugs in spurts for a good time, and it just sneaks up on 'em. Doesn't matter if your rich or poor, glamorous or glamourless, your life goes down the same rat hole. It's just some people disguise it better than others. Why even you, with all your education, could be flipped. If you give me 'nough time and the right stuff you'd be right here next to me."

I said nothing knowing how many doctors and nurses struggle with addictions.

"Everyday I have to fight the fight," Lester went on. "I know God is helping me, but I would like people to walk with me instead of avoiding me."

Shame welled up within me for my holier-than-thou attitude, for looking down upon Lester and his addiction, When in my own life there were the same failures and lack of self-control. A verse in Romans popped into my head:

*"You, therefore, have no excuse, you who pass judgment on someone else, for at whatever point you judge the other, you are condemning yourself, because you who pass judgment do the*

*same things." Romans 2:1 NIV*

"Forgive me Lester," I said. "You are right, I struggle with self-control, and depend on the Lord's mercy just as much as you. I can't tell you, how many times I have pleaded for God to overcome my deficiency of self-discipline and falling to temptation. Each time I feel like I have reached the limit of God's forgiveness."

"Yeah, I know that feeling," chimed in Lester. "It's all I can do to believe God will forgive me again. Dave told me it is all part of God's plan, that we become totally dependent on God by having to throw ourselves at the feet of Jesus, even when our bodies are screaming otherwise."

"Good ol' Dave," I murmured. I needed to hear that.

One day, Lester did not show for his appointment and we all knew why. The office staff would miss his toothless smile and the cheery laugh. He had become very special to everyone.

*"The thief comes only to steal and kill and destroy; I have come that they may have life, and have it to the full." John 10:10 NIV*

No one is beyond the reach of being entrapped by addictions, given time and repeated use we all would become enslaved. Not just drugs but also alcohol, pornography, gambling, and video gaming can become just as habit forming, Though on the physical level not as deadly, they can be just as enslaving to our spirit.

There is scientific evidence that addictions change our brain function. The neural pathways become geared to the compulsive behavior and it takes time and effort to repair the deep ruts these addictions cause. Obviously, the best course is prevention, but we all suffer from an ancient curse called temptation. This, combined with curiosity and rationalization, makes us all susceptible to becoming addicted. How many times have you told yourself: "I wonder what it would feel like?" Mix this with a rationalization like: "I will stop before it gets serious," or "It won't happen to me," and you are on the road to addictions. Therefore, we all need to realize we are not much different than the Lester's of life. By recognizing our own human frailty and weakness, we can encourage each other into healthy thinking and activities. That is the function of a good support group: to come alongside and urge one another in what is good, holding each other up in prayer.

> *"Finally, brothers, whatever is true, whatever is honorable, whatever is just, whatever is pure, whatever is lovely, whatever is commendable, if there is any excellence, if there is anything worthy of praise, think about these things." Philippians 4:8 NIV*

SECTION 3

# Seeds, Soil, and Hope

*"'A farmer went out to plant his seed. As he scattered it across his field, some seed fell on a footpath, where it was stepped on, and the birds ate it. Other seed fell among rocks. It began to grow, but the plant soon wilted and died for lack of moisture. Other seed fell among thorns that grew up with it and choked out the tender plants. Still other seed fell on fertile soil. This seed grew and produced a crop that was a hundred times as much as had been planted!' When he had said this, he called out, 'Anyone with ears to hear should listen and understand.'" Luke 8: 5-8 NIV*

But how do you know what type of soil you are? Is it based upon whether you relapse or not?

CHAPTER 9

# Hard Soil, Hard Consequences

My next patient I had known since his birth. Now eighteen he had been sent in by the court for evaluation following a DWI (Driving While Impaired).

> Every day, about thirty people in the United States die in alcohol-impaired vehicle crashes. Nearly one million people a year are charged with DWI, but the number of people who drive while impaired is estimated to be ten times that amount.

"What happened Jeff?" I said as I sat down on the exam room stool.

"Not much," Jeff shrugged. "I got pulled over coming home from a party. The cops said the car went over the center line a few times, but I think they were just looking to hit their ticket quota so they could loaf the rest of the night."

"Jeff, you can stop the charade, be honest," I said leaning forward hoping to break through his tough exterior. "This visit is about you. What did you ingest at the party?"

"Why should I tell you? I'm only here because the judge made me come," Jeff answered as he leaned back into the chair his arms folded across his chest.

"Look, you had a breath alcohol of 0.08 in the police report. So you can be honest with me about what else you took, or I'll order drug screening tests of your hair which will show drug use in the past six months. Then I'll tell the judge you were uncooperative."

Jeff shifted in his chair then shrugged, "Nothing much; the usual party stuff."

"Okay, how many drinks did you take at the party?"

"Who keeps track of that at a party?" he laughed. "I had a few Jello shots and some beer."

"Any drugs going around?"

"Oh, the usual party drugs, but I don't use any of them. I don't like how they make me feel."

"What does make you feel good?" I probed.

"I like weed mostly."

"So do you take it regularly?"

"I take it to relax after school. I take it at parties with alcohol because it gives me a nice buzz. A lot of people do marijuana, some have it prescribed. Why, I bet you have tried it too."

For adolescents using marijuana daily there is a 50% chance of addiction.

Twenty-five percent of those who begin abusing prescription drugs at age 13 or younger develop a substance use disorder at some time in their lives.

"Honestly, I haven't, but that does not affect the truth of the choice you face. You are looking for an excuse to use drugs, because you think everyone does it you think it is okay for you. This is not about how many others use drugs, or whether the drugs have medical indications. So tell me, why do you choose to take alcohol and marijuana?"

"Duh. I like the way it makes me feel," Jeff responded.

"Let me rephrase that for you. You use drugs to control the way you feel," I said.

"Sure, what's wrong with that?"

"I can tell you from the experience of others, this supposed control over your feelings turns out to be an evil trick. Instead of you retaining control, the drug slowly controls you and becomes the sole way you can feel any pleasure in life. Eventually, it even stops making you feel good, but you can't stop without slipping into depression and withdrawal. You no longer enjoy the simple things, sunshine after a rain, or the love of your family, because life becomes all about the drug."

Jeff rolled his eyes. "Yeah, well if you had my family you would choose to get drunk and use weed too."

"What would you change in your family relationships to choose them over alcohol and marijuana?" I said hoping to get him thinking in a new direction.

Jeff stopped to ponder his response, then spoke. "My family could never make me feel as good as weed does."

"Do you hear what you are saying? Life for you is not about family and enjoying the company of others, it has been high-jacked by the pursuit of a chemical high. Your friends don't come to your party to enjoy your friendship they come for the pleasure of getting high. Can't you see the trap you are in?"

"Back it up Doc. All I did was drive after taking a little alcohol and weed. It is not like I'm some crackhead living under the bridge."

"Circumstances may be different," I countered, "but the enslavement is the same—you will need a drug to keep from feeling sick or depressed. Be honest, do you enjoy being sober?"

Jeff sat there saying nothing, his expression signaled he had grown bored with our conversation. Not willing to give up yet, I plowed ahead, "I wish I could take you to the end of your life so you could look back and give yourself understanding of what is really important, like Scrooge in 'A Christmas Carol.' What would you say to yourself?"

"Nothing, this is stupid if you ask me," shrugged Jeff.

"Is there nothing left of you under this hard exterior?" I probed. "No feelings for real life, no glimmer of caring for others beyond yourself? Have the drugs already addled your brain?"

"What are you talking about?" Jeff said with irritation.

Drugs and alcohol negatively alter your thinking.

"Now you're sounding like my parents," Jeff complained.

MRI scans have shown structural changes in the brains of adolescents who are heavy users of alcohol and marijuana.

Ignoring his sarcasm I pushed on, "You hear only one thing about drugs and alcohol, a voice from within seducing you to eat at the trough of self-indulgence. So you go, small bites at first, but feeling only pleasure, you return more frequently feeding longer each time. Then one day you can't live without feeding at the pigsty you've made. The pleasure that enticed you at first has lost any gratification; instead, you must feed, or misery whips your body. There is no room for love, joy, peace, kindness and no self-control, for you have given over control to this foul appetite. Already I look and see your soul being eaten away, but all you can say is 'this is stupid'. No, to the contrary you are the fool…a beast going to the slaughter. Wake up!"

My eyes fixed on Jeff; he looked at me surprised by my outburst.

"Think about it, I'll see you next week," I said getting up. As I watched Jeff leave I prayed that God would break through his hard exterior.

*"This is the meaning of the parable: The seed is the word of God. Those along the path are the ones who hear, and then the devil comes and takes away the word from their hearts, so that they may not believe and be saved." Luke 8:11-12 NIV*

Jeff did not see his use of alcohol and marijuana as anything more than having a little fun. This denial of his problem hampers any chance of meaningful change. As the drug use progresses to addiction the denial becomes a means to hide the awful truth of what he has become.

I did not see Jeff again for six months. Then one day his name appeared on my schedule. Before entering the room my nurse whispered, "He looks awful."

"Jeff, it's good to see you, where have you been?" I said, trying to be as cheery as possible.

Jeff did not look up, his face buried in his hands, hair long and tangled. "I got caught driving with a suspended license and a BAC of 0.08. I had a deferred sentence from the previous DWI that the court reinstated. I am not in the mood for lectures—It's been hell."

"I thought your original sentence stood at 30 days in jail?"

"They tacked on five months cause I hit some old guy crossing the street."

"Oh, I'm sorry to hear that." I sat down and pulled the stool up close waiting for Jeff to speak.

"I never want to go back to jail. I'll kill myself before I go through that again."

"Then tell me, how can I help you?" Jeff paused for a long time and did not move.

"Jeff, you need to be honest with me," my voice broke the silence. "Mutual trust is the only way we can proceed; I will hold everything you say in confidence."

Again Jeff gave no response.

"Jeff, what do you hope for?"

"Hope?" He sighed with resignation. "My hope is oxycodone. I started snorting it in jail because I couldn't use weed and alcohol. At first it was just to feel good, you know, to cope with being locked up. But after a while, I started getting the shakes if I went too long without my medicine. In jail you end up doing things… horrible things just to avoid the sickness." Jeff looked at the floor to avoid my gaze. After a brief silence he went on. "Can't you understand you gotta help me, because if I fail the drug test with my PO (probation officer) they will lock me up."

"Jeff, what do you really want?" I said feeling Jeff's agony.

"What do you mean, 'what do I really want?'" Jeff looked irritated. "I want to stay out of jail and not be dope sick."

"And…" I asked trying to draw out more.

"Huh? Stop this guess-what-I'm-thinking and give me something that won't show up on the urine drug screen," responded Jeff.

He looked at me for the first time and on his left cheek I saw a jail tattoo. My heart ached for this boy I had known since his birth and now had wandered so far away.

"I hope you see the true prison you're in," I said praying for wisdom. "The obvious way to stay out of prison is by not taking any drugs, but we both know you relinquished that choice to the drugs a while back. Now your only choice is to figure out ways to hide your addiction. Can you see the pit you have fallen into?"

"Are you going to help me or not?" Jeff complained.

Not wanting to give up trying to get Jeff to face the truth I plodded on, "You came in wishing to get drugs to stave off withdrawal and slip past the urine test. But don't you ever hope you could really live the life God has always intended for you?"

"Hope?...Wishing upon a star went out with my childhood," Jeff derided.

"Hope is not words strung together into a wish, it is the direction you plot for living and depends on what you place your hope upon. Part of the curse of addiction is the drug becomes your hope to the detriment of everything else. So instead of hoping for Jesus in His fullness you hope to avoid withdrawal and stay out of jail."

"I asked God to help me back in prison, and it didn't work."

"Maybe you put your hope in the wrong thing. You were hoping for a miracle done your way, instead of hoping in Jesus, and His way."

"Yeah, yeah, yeah, whatever you say, Doc. But will you help me?"

"Yes, I will, but you must understand my goal is the life God wants for you, not something to allow you to continue in this wretched state."

"But I can't quit!" Jeff buried his head in his hands.

"All I ask is that you commit to trying," I encouraged.

"What am I supposed to say?" protested Jeff. "You're the one who controls the stuff."

"Let me frame the crossroads you face a little clearer. I don't control anything except how many pills I prescribe. It is you who must decide how much effort you put into the program. This is not a choice between using and not using drugs, that choice is long past. This is a choice to commit to trying, however long it takes."

Jeff sat there thinking for a long while then spoke, "I want to stop, but I'm scared I can't."

"I'll commit to helping you," I said. "If you commit to being helped."

"Okay," Jeff said quietly. "I'll try."

CHAPTER 10

# Building on Sand

*"Why do you call me, 'Lord, Lord,' and do not do what I say... But the one who hears my words and does not put them into practice is like a man who built a house on the ground without a foundation. The moment the torrent struck that house, it collapsed and its destruction was complete." Luke 6:46-49 NIV*

Dr. John Cody had many admirers in town. For over ten years he had worked caring for his patients and serving the community. He would often say about his medical practice, "I always want to do a little more for God." His skill as a doctor only propelled his popularity and demand for his consultation on difficult medical problems. He never said no to caring for patients regardless of the day or hour. I marveled at his detailed workups, vast knowledge of disease, and his dedication to medicine. If ever you were stumped over a diagnosis, Dr. Cody could be counted on for a detailed evaluation and plan.

He had it all, and that became part of the problem. He tried to be everything for everyone. His days were spent at the office with a packed patient schedule, and evenings rounding on hospital patients or doing consults. Unknown to anyone, this hectic pace began to take a toll, and to keep up he occasionally took Adderall (amphetamine) from medication samples he kept at his office. In time he began using them on a regular basis, but this introduced a new problem. The stimulant wouldn't let him fall asleep at night and he would be up at all hours. To counter the effect of Adderall, Dr. Cody began using Tylenol #3 (Tylenol plus the narcotic codeine) to come down and enable sleep. Soon the amount of Tylenol #3 for getting to sleep went up as Dr. Cody needed more and more drug to get any effect. This in turn caused him to use more amphetamine to wake up and be able to work. This vicious cycle of drugs began to be hard to keep under control. Rumors began to circulate in the hospital where he held the position of chief of staff, and in town where Dr. Cody served as an elder at the area's largest church.

One morning I had just finished a delivery. The hour being too late to go home for sleep, but too early to wake patients for morning hospital rounds, I elected to doze at the nurse's station.

"Ting" a call light went on for Mrs. Garner, one of my patients. She had a series of difficult interconnected medical problems. Attempts to gain control of one problem invariably led to a breakdown in another part of her body. Wondering what could be happening now, I got up and went down to her room to see what new calamity lurked. Fortunately, she had just rolled and accidentally hit the call button. I turned it off smiled at Mr. Garner, who looked up from dozing at his wife's bedside.

"No problem," I reassured him.

As I walked out Mr. Garner got up and followed me.

"Doctor Hufman can I speak to you," he said in a low whisper.

"Sure how can I help you," I responded.

"I don't want Dr. Cody consulting on my wife's care anymore," he said.

"Why, did something happen?"

"Last night he came in late to see my wife and his speech was slurred, then while writing in the chart he nodded off a few times. Something is wrong. He certainly shouldn't drive in that condition, let alone give medical care."

"Oh, I am sorry that happened. Maybe he was just tired."

"He wouldn't even look me in the eye when I asked him about it. No, I think there is something wrong."

I thanked Mr. Garner for telling me, and I promised to look into this immediately. Returning to the nurse's station I asked if anyone had seen Dr. Cody this morning. No one had, but they suggested checking the doctor's lounge.

"If Dr. Cody comes in during the night to see a patient, he will often just stay and sleep here," said one of the nurses. "If the door to the on-call bedroom is closed with the do-not-disturb card hanging on the handle, it's probably him. He usually gets up at seven to start morning rounds."

"Does he spend a lot of nights here?" I asked.

"Well,..." the nurse stopped, thought briefly, "Mmm, don't ask me, ask him," she said opening one of several charts before her.

"You were going to say?" I prompted.

"Nothing really, it is none of my business. I have to finish charting so I can go home, so please excuse me."

I went to the doctor's lounge and there on the closed door to the on-call bedroom hung the do-not-disturb sign.

I debated for a minute on whether to knock and rouse John. I decided to sit and wait. I had a number of charts stacked up needing telephone orders signed and discharge dictations to be completed. Plenty of work to occupy my time.

After twenty minutes, I heard some movement and muffled talking. Then the door cracked open and Dr. Cody slipped out closing the door quickly behind him.

"Good morning, catching up on old charts I see. They are a necessary pain I guess," Dr. Cody said in his usual affable manner.

"I need to talk with you," I said.

"Sure, but could we talk in the bathroom I really need to go."

"I can wait," I said.

"No, no, it's okay, we can talk in the bathroom as well as anywhere," said John.

I followed him into the bathroom He stepped up to the urinal. "Now, what's the problem."

"It's about Mrs. Garner."

"Yes, a very difficult case, I have dictated an extensive note on her and I will be happy to follow along with you on her treatment."

"Thanks, but Mr. Garner requests you not be involved."

"Why, is it something I said?" inquired John.

"It is more how you said it. He claims you were slurring your words and falling asleep during the work-up."

"Well, I may have been a little tired, but thanks to a little sleep I am rock solid now."

"If you are pushing yourself so hard that you are falling asleep during patient care, then you need to cut back and get more rest...don't you think?"

"Come on, we've been friends a long time; you know I would never jeopardize patient safety. Besides the Lord will renew my strength."

As John washed his hands, I noticed a slight tremor. He saw my gaze and as he left, shrugged with a chuckle, "Good thing I am not a surgeon."

John left the lounge, and I returned to my charts. Sitting down I noticed the on-call room door stood ajar and the do-not-disturb sign had been removed. I don't recall John going back and removing that sign. So on a whim I decided to check the room. The bedding laid disheveled at the foot on the floor, along with a few medical magazines. Quite a mess for house-keeping, I thought. I picked up the magazines and put them back on the end table. In the trash I saw a crumpled piece of notepaper with the hospital logo. Flattening the paper out it read, "chart review at 5" written in Dr. Cody's typical scribble. I threw it back in the trash and walked out to finish my charts and start hospital rounds.

Unknown to me, Mr. Garner had also made a complaint to the hospital administrator, and added that he thought Dr. Cody looked and acted like he had taken something. He didn't know what, but didn't want him near his wife.

The following morning the administrator stopped me in the hall and asked me to step into his office. I entered to see Nurse Langford, nursing supervisor, sitting pouring over the medical staff by-laws. She looked up and got right to the point. "My staff for weeks has felt Dr. Cody has been acting strange. At times, he is fast talking with a slight tremor and other times he nods off while writing orders. Then yesterday Mr. Garner made a complaint. That forces us to investigate this further."

"I am not sure how this involves me," I said.

"We've checked the by-laws for how to handle this," the administrator said. "As medical staff secretary you are to fill in when the chief of staff is unable to fulfill his duties."

"Wait, I was told you didn't have to do anything as secretary except read the minutes!"

"You need to do an exam," Nurse Langford shot back, "and obtain a urine specimen for drug screen from Dr. Cody, so we can determine what may be causing this behavior." She abruptly closed the notebook on her lap and added, "With Mr. Garner's complaint, I am worried that patient care is being compromised."

"Let me get this straight, you want me to go up to Dr. Cody and say 'The hospital wants you to submit for an exam and a drug screen?'"

"Yes," they both said in unison.

"All because of one patient complaint?" I protested.

"No, unfortunately there is more," Nurse Langford said in a doleful tone. "Jane Bower one of our night shift nursing aids has been seeing Dr. Cody,"

"You mean as a patient?" I asked. "How does that make any difference; besides, isn't personal information confidential?"

"It is until it affects patient care. I confronted Jane yesterday morning about being absent from the floor during her shift. The night supervisor had called her on it twice before, so this time she brought it to my attention, and that's how I came to speak with Jane Bower. As we talked, it struck me that she was acting odd, drifting during our conversation, not like the typical person coming off a night shift. So I asked her to give a urine sample for drug screening as per hospital staff guidelines.

She became angry and refused. I informed her that I had probable cause and a refusal could be considered a positive test. Because of that, I would have to put her on leave until the hospital could verify her fitness for duty. She became a little anxious and revealed she had been taking hydrocodone prescribed by Dr. Cody for menstrual cramps and headaches. I then asked to see the prescription bottle, or tell me what pharmacy I could call to get confirmation. She balked at first, but then told me that Dr. Cody gave her hydrocodone from his office supply."

"So, I'll tell John to stop giving out narcotics to patients," I said getting up to leave. "I am sure he doesn't want to get anyone in trouble. He's a good doctor, just a little too kind hearted is all."

"I hope you are right, but I am afraid there is more to the story." Nurse Langford motioned for me to sit down again. "I asked Jane to explain her absence from the floor yesterday morning about five. I mentioned that she had been seen entering the doctor's lounge where Dr. Cody had gone earlier to get some sleep. She became indignant and told me she was just retrieving a chart to double check a patients medication list."

My mouth went dry as I recalled the crumpled note that I had seen in the trash of the on-call room. I paused trying to weigh carefully what I should say. I didn't want to add gossip and unfounded rumors to this mess.

"I went to the doctor's lounge yesterday morning at about 5:30," I said. I explained finding the note in Dr. Cody's handwriting.

Nurse Langford sat for a moment and then said, "I have a hunch on what is going on, but you need to carry through with a drug screen and exam on Dr. Cody. I will pursue getting a drug screen on Jane Bower. If it is as I suspect, I'll put her on administrative reassignment until we get this cleared up. Oh, make sure you do an observed collection and preserve chain of custody in case this turns ugly."

Great, how am I going to pull this off especially on a friend.

I felt like some double agent, but this involved patient safety, and I knew I needed to proceed. The urine collection and exam had to be unannounced, so I decided to do it early in the morning when John had spent the night at the hospital. His next ER call night would be in two days. I tried to rehearse what I would say, but nothing sounded right so I decided to play it by ear.

CHAPTER 11

# The Collapse

I came to the hospital about 6 AM. The night nurse supervisor confirmed that Dr. Cody had gone to the on-call room at 2:30 AM, and should still be there. Lab had been alerted by the administrator about the need for confidentiality and chain of custody for the urine specimen. I then proceeded to the doctor's lounge. As expected, the on-call room had the do-not-disturb sign on the closed door. I debated whether to knock and get this over with but finally decided to give my friend the courtesy of sleep. I couldn't concentrate on charting so I just sat waiting and praying for wisdom. About 6:30 I heard some movement and decided John must be awake. So I went up to the door and knocked.

"John, it's Steve Hufman, we need to talk."

From behind the door came John's voice, "I can't right now but I'll meet you at the nurse's station in five minutes."

"No, I need to see you now."

"What in the world could be so important that it won't wait five minutes?"

"Just come on out and we'll talk about it." I said a little worried by all the stalling.

The door opened a crack I saw John peering out shirt unbuttoned and hair going every which-way.

"Can you at least let me get dressed," John said with growing anger.

"Sure," I responded trying to be cheerful.

"Then go sit down and I'll be out as soon as I get my pants and shoes on."

I turned to go sit down across the room, then thought, no something is wrong. As I turned back, John opened the door to step out. Behind him the light from the lounge lit up the form of Jane Bower frantically putting on her clothes.

John closed the door quickly. Seeing the shock on my face he said, "It's not what you think."

"I want you to give me a urine specimen. Nurse Bower can leave when we are in the bathroom." I handed him the container enclosed in plastic and held the door to the bathroom open waiting for him.

He took the bag, opened it, and headed for the toilet stall.

"It has to be an observed collection," I said.

"How can you call yourself a friend and put me through all this humiliation without even hearing me out?" John protested.

"Give me the urine specimen and we will talk."

"Well, you are going to make us stand here a long time because I used the bathroom just before you came in, and I find having someone stand there watching makes it difficult to relax. I must say I find you doing this to me most unkind and egregious."

"You think I take joy in this? You're the one whose actions are egregious." I said getting irritated with John's pomposity.

"Let's sit down and I'll explain how wrong these spurious allegations are," John said pulling himself together and stepping away from the urinal.

We went back into the lounge, Jane had long since left.

"Jane Bower is my patient. Though I don't have her express permission to share her medical treatment with you I am sure she will understand under the circumstances. I am seeing her for an ongoing problem with opiates that started with the reckless prescribing by another physician. I have been working with her to help her taper off."

"In the on-call room during the middle of the night?" I asked.

"Yes, for two very good reasons: she has a family and can't make appointments during the day. Her husband does not know of her opiate problem, and repeated appointments would make him suspicious. The other reason is she can't afford treatment so I meet with her here one or two nights a week to give her counsel and the pills she needs till our next visit."

"You know of course, what you are doing is illegal. With no documentation and giving her narcotics you could lose your license." I was not sure what to believe.

"I realize I have let my desire to help people take me into questionable areas, and I thank you for making me aware of the risk. Trust me, I will correct the deficiencies you have brought to my attention."

"You need to ask yourself if what you are doing is pleasing to God. As an elder of your church you should strive to keep things above reproach."

"Of course, that's important, but don't you see I am trying to serve God as best I can. Which is part of the reason for secrecy, all this is privileged information? You don't want to break patient confidentiality, and destroy her family by spreading spurious gossip, do you?"

"This is not the right way to treat addictions." I said shaking my head. "Does your wife know of these visits?"

"Well, well, well, look who is lecturing me on treatment of addictions. I think one of your patients recently died of a methadone overdose from a prescription you wrote. Why do you look at the splinter in my eye and not deal with the plank in your own?" John said with a sly smile.

At that moment the lounge door opened and Dr. Bell entered. "Sorry if I am interrupting but I have surgery scheduled." He grabbed some surgical scrubs and went into the bathroom to change.

"I think our conversation is over," Dr. Cody said as he got up and left.

Later that day, I met with the administrator and Nurse Langford and told them what happened in my meeting with Dr. Cody.

"My, he is smooth," Nurse Langford said. "But what he doesn't know is the night supervisor called me early this morning informing me that Jane Bower had been absent again. I came right in and caught Jane coming down the hall from the doctor's lounge. She had just finished tucking in her blouse, but had misaligned the buttons. I took her to my office, and we had a long talk."

"Does her story fit with Dr. Cody's?" I inquired.

"In many ways yes. She did admit to an opiate problem that started before she moved here. Initially, Dr. Cody tried a tapper, but soon her husband became angry over the cost and jealous about the weekly visits with Dr. Cody. That's when they switched to off-hour visits to coincide with when her husband worked at the mill. He eventually became suspicious and started calling home during breaks. If no one answered he would be abusive to her when he got home. So she came to work here as a nursing aid on night shift to get away from her husband and make it easier for her to see Dr. Cody. He then started surreptitiously giving Jane hydrocodone from his office, and hide the fact she was still seeing him. Even with this arrangement her fear and anxiety grew. That's when she started taking extra to help calm down. Dr. Cody told her he understood her anxiety because he sometimes used opiates to calm down after long stressful days. These night time sessions soon turned from counseling to sex, after which he would give her a one week supply. Soon, she became afraid that he wouldn't give her the pills unless they had intercourse. Even more worrisome to Jane is what her husband would do to Dr. Cody if he ever found out."

"This is worse than I could have imagined," the administrator groaned. "What do we do?"

"I think Dr. Cody needs to leave town for his own safety," said Nurse Langford.

"I know of a drug rehab program in Seattle tailored for physicians," I offered.

"But how do we get him in? He may not want to go," said the administrator.

"Oh, I think Dr. Cody will go when he understands what Mr. Bower might do if he learns of this affair," said Nurse Langford. "Besides, he will be forced to go when we report this to the state medical board, and we have to report it because it involves a patient."

"That is a plan for Dr. Cody, but what of Jane Bower? She can't work here in her current condition—she needs treatment. I am also worried what her husband will do to her if she seeks help," said the administrator.

"We need to set her up with the option of in-patient treatment with a strong social services aspect to work through these problems. Maybe we could have the social worker here at the hospital help Jane set something up and work out the financial hurdles." I said.

"We will work with Jane, and contact the state medical licensing board, and you,..." Nurse Langford nodded in my direction, "will talk with Dr. Cody and get him to go into treatment."

I dreaded that conversation, yet I also felt anger at being manipulated and wanted to confront him.

"Dr. Hufman," Nurse Langford broke into my thoughts. "We may also need your prescriptive help for Jane till she gets into treatment."

"We meet again tomorrow at noon to keep everything moving forward," the administrator said, looking at me.

I left, worried at what Mr. Bower would do if he should find out, and that put urgency to my meeting with John.

I went to Dr. Cody's office at lunch, when I knew he would not be seeing patients, and be alone catching up on dictation from that morning. I knocked on the partially open door to his office.

"May I come in?"

"What... are you here to try for another urine specimen?" he said eyeing me with suspicion.

"No, I am here to let you know Nurse Langford met with

Jane Bower, and we are notifying the state medical board about your affair with a patient and the inappropriate dispensing of narcotics. We are also telling them of your personal use of opiates."

John's jaw dropped. "Why are you doing this to me, are you trying to wreck my life? I thought we were friends, brothers in Christ. Shouldn't you be trying to help me instead of repeating small town rumors? What happened that you no longer believe me or give me the benefit of the doubt?"

"I admit I don't know everything, and your deception makes things even murkier. What I do know is the result of your activities you have led a patient who trusted you into worse addiction. Then used her weakness to commit adultery, potentially ripping apart both your families. The state medical licensing board will be investigating soon, and when Mr. Bower discovers what you have done, I am concerned for your safety. Now I think the best course of action is for you to seek help at the physicians drug rehab program in Seattle. Here is the phone number." I laid the number on his desk.

John wiped tears from his eyes as he tried to sift through all that his life had come to. "Don't you see, I just wanted to help people. To be God's instrument."

"You have helped people, and still can, but not when you're using drugs like hydrocodone, and not when you do things your own way instead of God's way," I said as I pushed the phone number closer.

"The drugs…" he slowly shook his head. "I only intended using them sporadically to help me keep going, you know, to help more people. Isn't that what God wants?"

"It's a deceptive bargain you made with drugs and now I am afraid they control you," I said. "John, face it, you need help. You can't do this alone."

"Where did it all go wrong?" John seemed to be talking to himself. "Drugs make you do things you never imagined you would do."

"Maybe the problem started when you put serving people above serving God. You tried to be the savior, instead of seeking His kingdom, His righteousness, His way."

"What am I going to do?"

"Well, you can start by doing what you know Jesus would have you do—ask for forgiveness, seek treatment, and end your affair with Jane Bower."

"You don't understand, I really do care about Jane—I love her."

"She was your patient you took advantage of her, that's not love."

"Yeah, well you're the one who needs to be showing a little more love. Isn't love supposed to be patient, and kind, and keeping no record of wrongs."

"You are so self-deceived I don't think you know what love is anymore. For everyone's sake you must stop any further contact with Jane and get yourself into drug treatment."

"I know I can help her, just give me a chance to straighten this out."

"John, listen to me! I am not going to argue with you. For the safety of your patients you must admit yourself into drug rehab. If you don't, we are ethically bound to report this to the state medical board and they will suspend your license. In the meantime, it is my duty to inform you that your hospital privileges have been suspended."

"But…"

"No buts! You need to call that number right now or you will force me to walk out that door and expose this ugly mess to the entire medical staff." I said. Under my breath I prayed, "Lord, have mercy; break through John's denial."

Dr. Cody picked up his phone and punched in the number. As I left, I heard him sob into the phone: "I think I need some help…"

In addictions, as with all things in life, the top priority

needs to be hearing God. Then with his help we can put what He says into practice.

*"But seek first his kingdom and his righteousness, and all these things will be given to you as well. Therefore, do not worry about tomorrow, for tomorrow will worry about itself. Each day has enough trouble of its own." Matthew 6:33-34 NIV*

CHAPTER 12

# Amy's Friends

Amy loved horses and the outdoors; she epitomized a Montanan—independent, strong willed, and loyal to her friends and family. She started off at a young age drinking with her older brother and his friends on weekends. It often became a contest of who could outlast the other in drinking. Amy hated to lose and soon found she could hold her alcohol better than most. Soon alcohol became an essential part of every activity and social occasion.

I first met her in the ER when her husband, Clayton, brought her in following a long weekend of drinking for her fortieth birthday. She had awakened that morning with a swollen belly and jaundice, looking very much like a squash balanced on two toothpicks. Her stomach pushed out from under her shirt, showing dark blue veins emanating out from a protuberant belly button. Her skin was stretched paper thin, a sickly yellow color with multiple sites of bleeding and bruising. The air she exhaled had the fetid odor of a musty attic. Her lab results returned confirming the sorrowful condition of her liver.

"You have cirrhosis of the liver," I explained. "That's a condition where the liver has been damaged to an extent that it can no longer keep up with normal liver functions. One such function is to get rid of bilirubin, a normal by-product of red blood cell breakdown; when that begins to back up in the blood, you develop jaundice. Also, the blood can't get through the damaged liver like it normally does, so it backs up causing fluid to build up in your abdomen called ascites. The bruising is from a deficient production of clotting factor in the liver. Putting this together with your history, I'd say you have severe alcoholic cirrhosis of the liver."

"Am I going to recover?" Amy asked.

"It depends on how much of the liver recovers from this last bout of alcohol consumption. You can function pretty well with only ten percent of your liver, but if you get much lower than that, your only option is a liver transplant."

"What! I am not that bad off, am I?" Amy, shot her husband a fearful look.

"We'll admit you to the hospital and get rid of the fluid. By letting your liver rest, hopefully in a few days it will bounce back. We'll repeat at some point and see how much your liver has recovered."

"Doc, you're scaring me," Amy shuddered.

"I'm sorry, but you should be scared," I replied. "You can't survive without a liver. You are teetering upon a life-and-death situation. I pray for your recovery, but you need to understand that alcohol induced cirrhosis is dose dependent. That means at some point the liver cannot tolerate another drink."

The next few days went well; her bloating cleared, and lab results returned to near normal levels. We had been talking all along about her liver not being able to handle any more alcohol. On the day of discharge, I reviewed what care she would need to take to maintain the liver function she had left.

"You should think of alcohol as poison, you could be one drink away from the tipping point with your liver." I warned.

"Don't worry, Doc. I am not going to touch any alcohol," she assured me.

"Yeah, I'll see to it," interjected Clayton.

"Clayton you need to stop too, or it will pull Amy back in at some point. I strongly suggest joining AA and avoiding any social gatherings where there is drinking."

Amy seemed uncomfortable with my last instruction. I continued hoping she would understand, "You both need to develop new friends who will encourage you to stay sober." I studied their faces trying to gauge how well they both grasped the gravity of Amy's cirrhosis.

Finally, Amy spoke up, "I can't tell my friends not to drink, and it doesn't seem fair to ask my husband to quit either. After all, I'm the one with the liver problem, not them."

"I really think the wise choice would be to stay clear of any alcohol," I reiterated, "or any situation which makes alcohol easily accessible. If you don't draw the line far enough away from the edge, you will slip back into old habits. The next drink could do you in."

"I'll quit for you," Clayton chimed in.

"No, I want to do this on my own. I'm the one who got into this and I have to be the one to get out." Amy sounded resolute in her decision to handle it herself.

"What about the Rodeo Club?" Asked Clayton looking toward me.

"What's the Rodeo Clu—"

Amy interrupted my question. "It's a bunch of horse lovers. We get together twice a month to have a little fun with our horses. Then afterwards we go to Little Joe's sports bar to talk and socialize. We are family."

Growing concern shadowed my face as I spoke, "I think you better not put yourself at risk of drink…"

"Oh Doc, I'll just tell them I can't have alcohol, they'll understand and not offer me any. After all, they're my friends."

A day later at discharge, I gave Amy instructions and told her to call and make an appointment in two weeks.

"What's the point of a follow-up visit?" she questioned with her usual cowboy bravado. "I either make it, or I don't."

Three months later, I gasped as I read her obituary in the paper. Sadly, the last line of the obituary summed up her life: "She died how she lived: with her friends, living life to the fullest. All her friends will be gathering this Saturday evening at Little Joe's for one last round in Amy's memory. Come share your favorite story. Cheers!"

Amy thought she could handle her addiction to alcohol, but fell back into it because she surrounded herself with people going in the opposite direction from where she needed to go. People with addictions have to accept the fact that their brains no longer can say, "NO" and hold to it. They need a complete shift in life patterns because traveling the paths that are associated with the addiction will lead them back into it. Amy let pride in doing it her way choke out seeking God's way.

For everyone the same can be said—you will become like those with whom you hang out. Families have to be clean and healthy if they want their child to be clean and healthy. All of us will be affected by the people and things we allow to surround us. Therefore, we must take care of what fills our life.

You can't withhold areas of your life from following God. Because, in doing so you are robbing yourself of His blessing.

*"Jesus replied, 'Blessed rather are those who hear the word of the God and obey it.'" Luke 11:28 NIV*

The 5th principle of Celebrate Recovery puts it this way:

Voluntarily submit to any and all changes God wants to make in my life and humbly ask Him to remove my character defects.

*"Happy are those whose greatest desire is to do what God requires." Matthew 5:6a TEV (GNT)*

SECTION 4

# Simple Gifts

*"And God confirmed the message by giving signs and wonders and various miracles and gifts of the Holy Spirit whenever he chose." Hebrews 2:4 NIV*

*"Praise the Lord; praise God our savior!*
*For each day he carries us in his arms.*
*Our God is a God who saves!*
*The Sovereign Lord rescues us from death."*
*Psalm 68:19-20 NIV*

CHAPTER 13

# Tiffany's Secret

"CPS (Child Protective Services) will take away my child if I don't get a letter from you stating that I don't have a problem with drugs or alcohol," Tiffany blurted out as soon as I entered the exam room.

Before me sat a beautiful young woman, attractively dressed and groomed, but in obvious distress. Not at all what I expected from the chief complaint scribbled in the chart: court ordered alcohol abuse evaluation, and fitness for caring for a child. Tiffany had come to me in the midst of a custody court battle with her ex-husband. It had become an ugly battle of accusations with lies and half truths slung about until no one knew the truth.

"It sounds serious, but why would anyone think you have a substance problem?" I said trying to coax more information without getting her more upset.

"My ex just can't stand me raising Teddy. He's an angry abusive man with a drinking problem. Since he can't be around Teddy, he would rather see my son in foster care, than happy with me. So I need you to tell the court I am okay."

"How can I honestly say anything since we have just met?" I asked, searching for clues as to uncover the truth. This young lady couldn't possibly have a problem with alcohol.

"I don't know--do lab tests or something, but I need that letter by next week."

"Okay, then let's begin. Have you ever done any drugs or used alcohol?"

"What kind of question is that? Everyone has, even you," Tiffany responded. Feeling uncomfortable she attempted to change the topic from her personal use. Her ploy to deflect attention to me, made me question my initial impression.

"Tiffany, you have come to me for assistance. I can only help you if you give me the truth, so tell me of your past use."

"I may have smoked a little weed in high school and gone to a few parties, but who hasn't?" she huffed.

"When was the last time you have used any substance, including alcohol?" I continued.

"I may have had a little wine with dinner last night just to unwind. Being a single parent to a 18 month old boy is not easy."

"How many drinks do you have in an average week?"

"I don't know, a few. Who keeps track of stuff like that?"

"Did you use any drug or alcohol during your pregnancy?" I asked softly trying to reassure her of my desire to help and not condemn.

"Maybe…I can't remember. I didn't keep a log book of my drinking; besides, an occasional drink is not going to hurt anyone." Tiffany averted my gaze.

"Tiffany, no one knows how much alcohol is safe during pregnancy. We do know that alcohol does affect the unborn child. Did you intend to drink during your pregnancy?" I could tell from her body language that inside she felt fear, but quickly covered it with indignation.

"I don't drink to get a buzz, if that is what you mean. I just use it when I get upset and need to calm down. Like you are doing to me right now!"

"I'm sorry if my questions upset…"

"Hey, I'm trying to be a good mom. Why are you saying all this...to make me feel bad?"

"Truly, I do not want to make you feel bad. I am just trying to find the truth about your use of alcohol. Does your pediatrician notice any issues with Teddy?"

"Teddy's a little hyperactive," she sniffled and blew her nose. "But the doctor says we need to wait till he is older to determine if he needs treatment."

"Did you mention to your doctor that you took alcohol

during the pregnancy?"

"Hey... what is this? Are you going to write the letter or not?"

"I want to see your child stay with you, but I have to be honest with the court, and that hinges on you being forthright with me."

"Okay, ask me and I will be as honest as I can. I have nothing to hide."

> The screening CAGE questionnaire is one of many aids for discerning who may have a problem.
>
> Have you ever felt you should Cut down on your drinking?
>
> Have people Annoyed you by criticizing your drinking?
>
> Have you ever felt bad or Guilty about your drinking?
>
> Have you ever had a drink first thing in the morning to steady your nerves or to get rid of a hangover (Eye opener)?
>
> Yes, to one or more of these questions may signal a problem.
>
> Caution: this is only an aid to determine who might need further evaluation. Similar screening questions exist for other addictions.

"Have you ever felt you should cut down on your drinking or drug use?"

"Sure, with my pregnancy, but everyone does."

"Have people annoyed you by criticizing your drinking or drug use."

"Oh, come on, what person doesn't get flack from their parents?"

"Have you ever felt bad or guilty about your drinking or

drug use?"

"There was once when I got smashed at a party and woke the next morning unsure what had happened. I couldn't believe I had been so stupid to drink that much."

"Have you ever drunk or used drugs first thing in the morning to calm your nerves or get rid of a hangover?"

"Are you kidding? Mornings and me don't get along, I need coffee not a drink."

With much care and concern I said, "Judging by your answers I think you may have a problem with alcohol."

"What! My answers make me an alcoholic?"

"I am not saying that, but I do think it is a possibility. Tell me how many times during your pregnancy did you promise yourself not to drink?"

A shadow came over Tiffany's face and her anger turned to remorse. She sat there crying with her face buried in her hands.

"Don't let them take Teddy from me. I have tried to do the best I can. I had an abusive father and married young just to get away. Then, turns out the guy I married drank and beat me as much as my old man. When I got pregnant, the abuse got worse, he called me all sorts of names."

"I am sorry to hear that," I said.

"I feel like such a failure," she sobbed.

I gave her a Kleenex and after a pause to blow her nose she went on, " I tried not to drink during my pregnancy. I even promised God. But things just fell apart; my ex drank and beatings were unbearable. I had to call the police a few times. Finally, I filed for a divorce and got a restraining order. Drinking became a way to make it through the stress of those days."

She took the box of tissues and went through a few more, sobbing, "I need Teddy! Can't you see how much I need him?"

Silently I prayed, "Lord, help this poor mother and help me know what to do."

She went on, "Now that I know I might lose Teddy, I have to drink just to cope with guilt. Yes, I've made some bad choices, but if they take my baby away, they might as well shoot me. You have to help me!"

> In the US over 40,000 babies are born each year with Fetal Alcohol Spectrum Disease. One recent study showed that 1-5% of school children suffer from FASD. In the case of opiates and pregnancy every 15 minutes a child is born in opioid withdrawal.

"I know you love Teddy, but continuing to drink is not going to be in your child's best interest. I want to help you find another way of dealing with your fears and guilt. Drowning your sorrows with alcohol does nothing to solve the problem, but only makes it worse. Instead, if you let the guilt lead you to God's forgiveness and asking Him for help, then in reality, the guilt becomes a tool for healing."

"Forgiveness?" Tiffany began to wail. "How can anyone forgive me when I can't forgive myself? I have broken so many promises to God. Worst of all, how can a mother forgive herself for doing what I've done to my son?"

"It is the same for all of us, when we face the truth about ourselves. The guilt can be crushing, but there is mercy and forgiveness with God. Here, listen to this Psalm." I reached for my Bible and began to read.

*"If you, O Lord, kept a record of sins,*
*O Lord, who could stand?*
*But with you there is forgiveness;*
*therefore you are feared.*
*I wait for the Lord, my soul waits,*
*and in his word I put my hope." Psalm 130:3-5 NIV*

Tiffany sat, tears streaming down her face. "Do you really

think there is hope for Teddy and forgiveness for me?"

"God is waiting for us to put our hope in Him instead of ourselves," I shared. "He is faithful even when we are faithless. I believe it for myself. I know His love is there for you."

"But I used alcohol during the pregnancy and hurt my Teddy. Can God ever forgive me for that?"

"I know God's mercy is great, and that He loves you and Teddy. You can trust that His love will see you through whatever hardship lies ahead. Have you ever heard the 23rd Psalm?"

"Yeah, I had to memorize it for my confirmation class." Tiffany paused to reflect. "I guess I didn't pay much attention."

"It says in verse 4: 'Even though I walk through the valley of the shadow of death, I will fear no evil, for you are with me.'"

"I wish I could believe that," she said with a tinge of remorse.

"God put it there for us to pray, I think He means it. That is where faith comes in."

"What about the letter for the court?"

I looked her straight in the eye. "I can't tell the court you are clean and sober, but if I tell them you are actively involved in a recovery program I would think they'll let you keep your child with supervision."

Tiffany considered the difficult road ahead her face clouded with fear, "How am I going to make it raising Teddy when I couldn't stay sober before?"

"You need God's help."

Tiffany struggled with the prospect of added stress of raising Teddy. A light seemed to brighten her countenance.

"I just remembered something else from confirmation class," she smiled as she spoke.

"What's that?" I inquired, wondering where she was going.

"Immanuel, means God is with us," she said. "If God gave us that name for Jesus, maybe it really does mean he wants to go with us, helping us through our problems."

As Tiffany left, she looked back at me and said with a tinge of hope, "I don't need to fear, for somehow Immanuel is with me."

"That 'somehow' is all God's doing, so you can count on it." I said. Then, as she disappeared around the corner I whispered, "Lord, thank You."

Hope for healing becomes the key ingredient to allowing someone to break free of addiction. Denial and rationalizations are no longer necessary to avoid facing the truth of enslavement to drugs, because with real hope the power of God is at work to bring about your healing from this terrible scourge.

*"The rain and snow come down from the heavens*
*and stay on the ground to water the earth.*
*They cause the grain to grow,*
*producing seed for the farmer*
*and bread for the hungry.*
*It is the same with my word.*
*I send it out, and it always produces fruit.*
*It will accomplish all I want it to,*
*and it will prosper everywhere I send it.*
*You will live in joy and peace.*
*The mountains and hills will burst into song,*
*and the trees of the field will clap their hands!*
*Where once there were thorns, cypress trees will grow.*
*Where nettles grew, myrtles will sprout up.*
*These events will bring great honor to the Lord's name;*
*they will be an everlasting sign of his power and love." Isaiah 55:10-13 NLT*

Jesus is the focus of our hope. The Great Physician, gives us life today and He is the assurance of God's goodness, love, and power for all our tomorrows. Most wonderful of all—this happens by God's power not ours.

*"We have this hope as an anchor for the soul," Hebrew 6:19 NIV*

*Our hope is this: "Jesus Christ in you, the hope of glory." Colossians 1:27 NIV*

*"What, then, shall we say in response to this? If God is for us, who can be against us? He who did not spare his own Son, but gave him up for us all—how will he not also, along with him, graciously give us all things?" Romans 8:31-32 NIV*

There is one thing to remember—you have to take this hope in God and let it grow. Jesus spoke about this in Luke 8, the Parable of the Sower:

*"As for what fell among the thorns, these are the ones who hear; but as they go on their way, they are choked by the cares and riches and pleasures of life, and their fruit does not mature. But as for that in the good soil, these are the ones who, when they hear the word, hold it fast in an honest and good heart, and bear fruit with patient endurance." Luke 8:14-15 NRSV*

Patient endurance is an attribute not many people have in abundance, yet it is vital in a recovery program. This is where a support group and mentor come in. Together they are stronger than any one individual, and together they can hold on to one another, encouraging growth into the fullness of what the Lord has in mind.

The first step in talking with someone who is using drugs is to help them to understand what or whom their hope is in—whom they are serving. Real hope in God allows you to break through all the denial because you no longer need to hide from the truth.

*"Therefore, there is now no condemnation for those who are in Christ Jesus." Romans 8:1 NIV*

Believing this about yourself can sometimes be difficult because of all the negative thoughts that pop up. That is why God sent the Holy Spirit to help us understand the truth.

*"But I will send you the Advocate—the Spirit of truth. He will come to you from the Father and will testify all about me." John 15:26 NLT*

To sift through and cleanse all the negative junk we have collected, there is even a prayer for that:

*"Search me, O God, and know my heart;*
*test me and know my anxious thoughts.*
*See if there is any offensive way in me,*
*and lead me in the way everlasting." Psalm 139:23-24 NIV*

CHAPTER 14

# Shaken by God

"I have never seen him this bad before." Jack had brought in his old drinking buddy, Fred, to the emergency room with the shakes. They were neighbors and friends, both retired from the lumber mill. Fred had lost his wife four years ago and had been on a long drunk ever since. When Jack stopped in to check on him he found him on the kitchen floor shaking and screaming about insects crawling all over him. According to Jack, Fred's place smelled of urine and his wife's cat. Jack had called the ambulance, and stood by now ready to help his friend.

When I walked into the ER the odor made me want to stop breathing and turn around.

"Doc, you need to help save Fred. He's been depressed about his wife Carol's death from cancer and trying to forget with a bottle. I promised her before she died I would take care of Fred and get him into the Lord's kingdom." Jack looked at me then gazed with worry at his friend shaking on the gurney. He then took off his hat and began to pray with a booming voice as if volume made the words more powerful. "Jesus, give Doc wisdom and pull Jack out of the DTs. Please Lord, don't let him die before he comes to know You. I know You love his wife, Carol, and she is with You now. Well, she had been praying for both of us until the day she died. You answered her prayer about me, so now please touch Jack's life and heart with the power of the Holy Ghost. Please, transform Fred's life like You did mine. In Jesus name amen."

Jack's tremor seemed to diminish slightly, but agitation now engulfed him and he begin thrashing about. Restraints where placed and Librium administered to calm him down and begin treating the DTs. Suddenly he began crying "Carol…Carol… why? Please, someone put me out of my misery. I don't want to live!"

"Has he ever had the delirium tremens before?" I asked trying to assess how serious this might be, for I knew of people dying from alcohol withdrawal. I had assisted in managing patients with DTs during my training and knew firsthand how rough this could become, but that played out in a regular detox unit at the VA hospital; here I was on my own without help.

"Yeah, about four months ago he had been drinking real regular, but ran out of booze the next day Fred got the shakes. I tried to get him to come to the hospital and dry out, but then another friend gave him a bottle of whiskey, and he's been on a bender ever since." Jack glanced with apprehension at his friend.

"Our hospital doesn't have an ICU to help get him through this, so we are going to have to ship him out," I said.

"I know Fred, and he won't stay where he doesn't know the people. You've heard him. He wants to die, but with God's help I know you can get him through this. Please, don't send him off. I'll stay with him till he's better, whatever it takes. I'll stand watch and be praying the whole time. I just know God's gonna do a miracle."

I looked at Fred, and by this time the Librium started to calm him a bit. He looked up at me and said, "Either help me here or send me home, but I ain't going to anywhere else, Doc."

We put Fred in a room nearest the nurses station, and Jack true to his word stayed with Fred. His booming prayers where heard by everyone at the nurses station. Other times he would read aloud from the Bible, telling Fred about forgiveness, and how much Jesus loved him.

After three days of up and down withdrawal symptoms, the worst of Fred's agitation subsided, and I finally saw him smile in sweet release from the DTs. On the morning of the fourth day I came into the room to give Fred the discharge instructions. Jack and Fred were praying with fits of laughter, oblivious to me.

"Uhmm, sorry to intrude. I just need to give you some discharge instructions."

"You're not intruding. We've just been thanking God for you and the nurses, but most of all for the power of Jesus to heal."

"Well, you're over the withdrawal but you still will be battling cravings for alcohol. I want to see you in the office in two days to go over your recovery plan. Obviously, you can't drink anymore, period. So, when you get home clean out anything that even smells of alcohol."

"Oh, I'll make sure of that," chimed in Jack.

"How do you plan to stay sober?" I asked. "I can prescribe Antabuse that will make you sick if you take any alcohol."

"No thanks Doc, I'm going to be attending AA with Jack. But the most important thing is Jesus is in my heart. I'm healed by the grace of God and don't want to touch another drop. Carol's prayers for me have been answered. Hallelujah!"

"That's great," I said, trying to hide my skepticism. "But you may have some fairly strong cravings, or difficult times when you want a drink. What is your plan then?"

"I can call on Jack any time, we live real close. What's most important is I know God loves me and wants to help me live for Him—that's the real miracle of the last few days. I have been forgiven and washed clean by Jesus. I'm sure Carol is praising God, for once I was lost but now I'm found. I was blind with alcohol, but now I see." Fred smiled and slapped me on the back. "Thanks for helping me." Then Fred looked me in the eye, "If there is anything I can do to help you, let me know."

"I'm just happy you made it through this," I said.

"Isn't God good," said Jack. "Pray with us, Doc," and he put his arm around me and Fred and began: "Thank you Jesus..."

Fred never touched alcohol again and became a community leader in helping others trapped by addictions. I find it amazing how God takes a washed up old drunk, dries him out and then makes him a beacon of light to others. Both Jack and Fred were amazing stories of God's grace. Sometimes people wonder why God doesn't heal everyone like he did Fred. I can only tell you what Fred told me. "In the end, it is all about God. You have to believe He is God, and that He loves you and wants to set you free. He gives each of us gifts, not all the same, so we each have an important role to play in His kingdom."

I need to review and renew my trust in God all the time. If I don't, pride starts to sneak in. That's why the most important gift of all is redemption in Jesus. Washing in His grace daily, letting Jesus redeem my day new and fresh. Part of that is choosing to believe He loves me in spite of my feelings about myself or circumstances. When my pride causes me to doubt God's love and the way He is doing things. That's when I force myself to kneel and pray till it finally sinks in—"He is God, and He loves me, and He knows what He is doing."

I have had to reflect upon Fred's words many times when things seem to be going wrong. "Lord, You are God, I am not, I want to do it your way not mine. Please forgive me and help me." This prayer has its greatest impact when we understand how much God loves us and desires to help even the most rotten scoundrel.

SECTION 5

# God Wants to Heal

No matter how many times we mess up, God is waiting to forgive us and wants to be with us. This truth is difficult to accept, for we feel so worthless, but even here God wants to help. The Bible has a story of a liar and cheat in whom God demonstrates His mercy and love.

> *"Then Jacob made a vow, saying, 'If God will be with me and will watch over me on this journey I am taking and will give me food to eat and clothes to wear so that I return safely to my father's house, then the Lord will be my God.'" Genesis 28:20 NIV*

This is an absurd bargain Jacob offers to God. Jacob has swindled his brother, Esau, lied to his father, Isaac, and is a coward at heart. Jacob should be punished for his life not be rewarded. Yet here Jacob is making a vow with God and God agrees. This helping of Jacob has nothing to do with Jacob's character, or any appealing quality. It can only be because God wants to help Jacob. This is exactly how it is for the worst addict—they have lied and cheated their family and friends to the point no one trusts them, or even wants to be around them. They have squandered any redeeming virtue, yet God steps in and says "I want them."

> *"And I pray that you, being rooted and established in love, may have power, together with all the saints, to grasp how wide and long and high and deep is the love of Christ," Ephesians 3:17-18 NIV*

CHAPTER 15

# Near Death

Alexi lived on the streets of Vinnytsya, Ukraine, doing anything and everything to get more heroin. That is all he lived for, but it was hardly a life. On the street they called it "killing time with heroin until it kills you." For Alexi, heroin or death became all he had to look forward to. After years of using drugs, Alexi had gone through all the usual spots for injecting heroin. Now, since he could find no veins for his needle, he began injecting heroin under the skin of his legs. They call this skin popping. These sites frequently become infected, causing pus draining ulcers, and Alexi had many such sores over his body.

The Ukrainian police had picked up Alexi for burglary, and after one day in jail he suddenly became delirious with chills and fever. The police checked Alexi and saw red streaks running up his legs from multiple infected ulcers. They had seen this before and knew Alexi did not have long to live. They couldn't take him to the hospital, for they would refuse to accept an infected drug addict. If he died in the jail, no one wanted to do the paper work necessary for disposing the body, so the police put Alexi in the transport van intending to dump him in some alley. On the way one officer remembered a church that worked with addicts and alcoholics. "We'll take him there, and they can deal with the body."

The van sped across town. They needed to dump him before he died or they would be stuck with the body. When they got to the church, they backed up to the door. "Not even God will want this one," the officers laughed as they flung Alexi on the front steps of the church, pounded on the door and took off like kids playing a prank.

This happened to be the evening of the church's all night prayer vigil. The congregation heard the van pull up, a rustling, followed by a bam bam bam on the door. Some men went to investigate and found Alexi unconscious in a crumpled pile on the doorstep. Hauling him in, they put Alexi on a cot at the back of the church and started to wash his infected wounds and use cool compresses to ease the fever. At the same time, the rest of the church prayed for Alexi. When morning came, Alexi still hung on to life. His raging fever had eased, and quiet breathing replaced his incessant groaning. The church's prayers moved from pleading to praise for the wonderful miracle taking place before their eyes. Over the next three days Alexi slowly took food, and had the strength to sit up. The congregation took turns ministering to him, each one telling Alexi of God's wonderful miracle to save and give meaning to his life.

"Alexi, God loves you… Jesus healed you and He wants you for his child… God has saved you for better things."

Alexi had never heard such strange talk of God loving him, but he knew he should have died. In fact, Alexi knew he deserved death for all the terrible things in his life, but here he laid being cared for by strangers. Alexi realized there could be no other answer as to why he lived—God loved him. "Jesus loves me," echoed over and over in his mind until it sank in. "Thank you Jesus, I should be dead but you saved me… You really must love me… I do not deserve this, but thank you… forgive me for I am a wretched man… You have redeemed me, please free me from my addictions and help me live for you."

It took weeks for Alexi to gain enough strength to stand and walk. During that time he had people reading to him from the Bible and teaching him to read for himself. To everyone's surprise his mind retained long passages of scripture and he started to share the verses with others.

"Look here," Alexi would say to anyone who would listen. "The Lord wants to give me grace and compassion: *'Yet the Lord longs to be gracious to you; he rises to show you compassion. For the Lord is a God of justice. Blessed are all who wait for him!' (Isaiah 30:18)* His word tells me to wait for Him. That He will tell me what I should do."

Over the months Alexi felt God had a special calling for his life—to minister to other addicts, and preach the good news of Jesus, the Great Physician who had miraculously healed him.

Alexi's whole family heard about his miraculous healing. But when they saw first hand the change in Alexi, they became convinced of God's power. If Jesus could take the useless life of a dying street addict and give him a new life, He truly must be the Christ and Savior of the world. Many joined Alexi in praising God and worshiping at the feet of Jesus. News of Alexi's healing spread through the streets, and many addicts came to see for themselves if they could be healed. Many joined Alexi in declaring the praises of Jesus, who called them out of darkness into his wonderful light.

As unbelievable as it seems I know the truth of this story because I stood on the banks of the Southern Buh River and witnessed Alexi baptize his family and many others rescued from the clutches of drugs and alcohol. That Sunday afternoon the heavens seemed to open in glorious praise to the Lord Jesus. Many transformed lives became proof that God wants to save us even when we are all but dead, and worthless.

There is one question that keeps popping up. If God wants to help us conquer our addictions, why doesn't he perform a miraculous healing in everyone? No one knows the answer, but what we do know is God loves us more than we can comprehend. He has shown His love for us in sending Jesus to die for us while we were His enemy lost to addictions. That fact is what holds us through all the horrible times. Still, some people discount Alexi's story as made up, but what they are really doubting is the love of God.

There are a few things to keep in mind before you question God's love and his desire to save:

1.) We cannot see what God sees, nor are we privy to the whole story.

2.) We cannot impugn God's wisdom and love without putting ourselves in judgment of God, and that is contrary to what you need—which is having Christ dwell in your heart through faith. Therefore, I encourage you to persevere in prayer and trust God's redeeming love, and let that anchor your soul.

> *"But do not forget this one thing, dear friends: With the Lord a day is like a thousand years, and a thousand years are like a day. The Lord is not slow in keeping his promise, as some understand slowness. He is patient with you, not wanting anyone to perish, but everyone to come to repentance." 2 Peter 3:8-9 NIV*

May God give us all power to grasp how much He wants to fill our need.

> *"...So that Christ may dwell in your hearts through faith. And I pray that you, being rooted and established in love, may have power, together with all the saints, to grasp how wide and long and high and deep is the love of Christ, and to know this love that surpasses knowledge—that you may be filled to the measure of all the fullness of God." Ephesians 3:17-18 NIV*

CHAPTER 16

# God Still Cares When We Do Not

"What's the use?" said Sam. "I have lost everything, including my soul."

Sam had been sent in for addiction treatment under court orders. He sat in my office a bundle of self-loathing and sorrow.

"I'm tired of trying. It's hopeless. Even if I kick my habit, I have no life left to go back to."

"I disagree," I responded. "You can still live a meaningful life. Even this day can have purpose—the start of a new beginning."

"That's easy for you to say, Doc, but you don't know my past. It's more evil than you can imagine, and I hate to think what my future holds. I have nothing to look forward to except death, and even there I failed twice already."

"Are you contemplating trying to kill yourself now?" I inquired.

"Well, if I don't get what I need, that might be my only option," Sam said holding his hands together to quiet the shake.

"It is not right for you to use threats of harm to get what you want. Besides, we both know if I don't give you drugs you can get them elsewhere," I said trying to figure out how to proceed.

"Wrong," he said pulling up his pant leg exposing an ankle monitoring bracelet. "You think they put this on me because I'm good? The probation officer can track me. If I go anywhere I shouldn't they'll send me back to jail. I just got out from five years behind bars for sexual assault on a minor. Do you have any idea what happens to people in jail for crimes against kids? No, you don't want to know, for even if I told you the gruesome details, it's nothing like going through it. I am telling you, Doc, I ain't going back there."

He paused to let these awful memories churn inside. Sam rolled up his sleeves revealing on his arms the most obscene tattoos of Satan I have ever seen. The ink camouflaged his injection sites by making them stars.

"This is what prison made me." He spit out. "I wish I were dead, but I don't have the guts for that so I take drugs to forget. Don't take that away from me or I will..." Sam's voice tapered off into thought.

"Or what?" I prompted.

Our eyes locked. I could see anger, pain, and fear surging about in his stare. Finally he spoke, "I will go to hell in a blaze of blood and gore, then you'll wish you'd helped me with what I need."

My mind whirled trying to gauge the danger of this moment and what to do next.

"I see you have great sadness over the fact your life has been filled with pain and evil of every type," I said trying to summarize and gain time. The second principle of Celebrate Recovery popped into my mind and I said it out loud, "Blessed are those who mourn, for they shall be comforted."

"What are you talking about?" questioned Sam. "I don't go for that religious stuff. If there is a God, He abandoned me a long time ago."

I continued, "The principle goes on to encourage us to earnestly believe that God exists, that you matter to Him and that He has the power to help you recover."

"Yeah, well, it's a little late, as you can see by my tattoos. To me, God is dead...or maybe it is more like I'm dead." Sam looked dejected as he said these words.

"We are all walking dead," I said trying to get through to Sam. "But God, in His love, found a way to bring us back to life in him."

Sam appeared to be battling inside—caught between wanting to believe, and the reality of his miserable life enslaved by drugs and darkness. Finally he spoke, "Doc, I am as good as dead, and no amount of religious talk will change that."

"I'm confident that God can do a miracle in you if you let him," I said looking at Sam for some clue of softening. After a long pause I asked, "May I pray for you?"

"Ah… sure," Sam said taken by surprise at my request.

"Lord, help Sam sense how much You love him. That the power of Christ's resurrection from the dead is there for him, to give hope where there is no hope and bring life where there is only death… Amen."

"So, will you give me some drugs?" asked Sam.

"I will help you get off of drugs," I replied. "But I won't just give you drugs."

Sam stood up, cussed, and walked out, not looking back. On his way out he screamed obscenities about my care to the staff and patients in the waiting room. Pushing over a potted plant at the entrance, he left leaving behind startled patients and staff. Later, he filed a complaint against me with the hospital administrator and the state medical board. I never heard from him again.

~

This may seem like an odd story to tell in a section concerning God's desire to meet our desperate need, especially because I have no idea what happened in Sam's life. I will say that the story is not complete and we will not know its conclusion until we stand before the throne of God.

Sam's visit with me was not an accident, but part of God reaching out to touch Sam's life and rescue him from the evil of this world. Sam's reaction to hearing of God's love, and the power of the resurrection of Christ, speaks of the ongoing spiritual warfare in this world. To deal with addictions, you must also deal with the spiritual.

For those who disapprove of my praying for Sam, and feel it messed up an opportunity to help Sam deal with his addictions, I have no defense. I wanted to help, but Sam didn't see it that way. Even now, I pray for Sam and ask the Lord to not let my clumsiness hinder this patient's recovery. For those working with people caught up in addictions there is a daily need to ask Jesus to redeem your thoughts and actions—to not let your mistakes cause injury, but somehow bring healing. You will find there is this dilemma in trying to help someone, when to be firm, and when to yield, when to stand back, and when to intervene, when to call out infractions, and when to let it go. You constantly second guess yourself when things seem to fall apart. In these circumstances all you can do is pray for discernment and trust that God will use your bumbling for His glory. For Sam, I earnestly hope and trust that in the end, God's love will prevail. For God so loved the world that he wants to meet our desperate need, even for someone as bent as Sam, or as bumbling as me.

*"If we are faithless,*
*He will remain faithful,*
*for He cannot disown himself." 2 Timothy 3:13 NIV*

*"Jesus Christ is the same yesterday and today and forever."*
*Hebrews 13:8 NIV*

CHAPTER 17

# A Promise to the Seeker

"You know the biggest problem with drugs?" Kyle said during one of his visits for addiction. "I mean besides dying from an overdose." At twenty-five years old Kyle had dropped out of college and burned through three jobs, and now worked part time at a mini-mart. He had a girlfriend, but she threatened to kick him out if he didn't get off drugs, which is what brought him into my office for Suboxone treatment.

"Tell me," I encouraged.

"The pursuit of more drugs becomes all you ever do. The only thing you can think about is: 'How am I going to get my next hit.' That thought keeps growing in your brain until everything else gets pushed aside. I'm telling you it's a beast you don't want to meet. You spend your life tiptoeing around, trying not to awaken the dragon, but it always awakens and bites as soon as your last hit begins to fade."

"Oh, I understand it's a major problem in addictions," I said wondering where Kyle was leading.

"No, you don't have the least bit of understanding. No one who hasn't gone through it realizes the horrible power of drugs. How it drives you to sacrifice everything to keep it satisfied. It's a relentless and all consuming monster that won't quit gnawing at you until you give it what it wants."

"Are you making an excuse for using?" I asked. "Sounds like you're deflecting responsibility for a choice you continue to make."

"See there, you're just like the rest. You have all these cheesy answers, but do not understand the problem. Do you think people <u>choose</u> to live on the street, selling everything they have, including their bodies, just for another fix? People understand someone who is starving and steals a loaf of bread because everyone has experienced hunger. But when it comes to drugs, they get on their high horse and spout nonsense because they have never been there and met the monster. It colors every decision every moment of the day. Like being too close to a burning fire. You must put it out, or back away. You can't just sit there and force yourself to think some pleasant thought."

"Good analogy," I said. "That's a common problem, of being unable to resist what is wrong. It is the first step of a 12-step program and the first principle of Celebrate Recovery: 'Realize I'm not God; I admit that I am powerless to control my tendency to do the wrong thing and that my life is unmanageable.' You won't seek help unless you admit you need help. But just any help won't do, what you need is help that is stronger than your addiction. This enslavement to darkness is not only found in drug addiction, but afflicts everyone in various ways. For we all like sheep have gone astray."

"Spare me the platitudes," Kyle protested. "You're sounding like some TV preacher."

"I agree with you that the truth can sound trite, but that doesn't make it any less true," I shrugged. "We all have problems that plague us, it's just that many maintain their denial and thus avoid facing the awful truth."

"Let me get this straight," said Kyle. "You're telling me everyone struggles with something?"

"Yes."

"What do you struggle with?"

"I have multiple things that keep me seeking the Lord's compassion and help."

"So tell me."

"If I thought it would truly help you I would tell you, but at this juncture I worry it would only sidetrack us from you dealing with your addiction. Also, there is the real chance you might be tempted to use it as another excuse to continue using drugs. I will tell you I have shame and need God's grace to live each day for Him."

"So if everyone has a similar problem, how can God condemn me for what no one, including you, can keep from doing?" asked Kyle.

"He loves us, and it's that love that condemns the ugliness that enslaves us. He won't overlook anything that keeps us from being all that we were created to be. Does not the loving mother wipe the snot off the nose of her child?"

"I wish my problem was just a little snot. You can't put drug addiction in the same ballpark as a child with a runny nose."

"I didn't mean to trivialize your problem. It's an analogy to help you understand God's desire is to make us completely clean. Even from hatred, lying, pornography, anger, the list goes on and on. Everything that is not of God needs to be forgiven and wiped clean."

"If only it were as easy as wiping my nose," said Kyle.

"There is no 'easy' when it comes to restoring us. It required Jesus to die in our place, and now requires us to have faith in Him, even when every part of our body is screaming otherwise. Trusting God is a daily thing and often it feels like you are not making any progress, but you have to trust that God knows what he is doing and will hold on to you through the tough times."

"Someone trying not to lie is not on the same level as drug addiction and fighting withdrawal," Kyle protested. "Drugs grip so tight you have no breath left for living. They screw up your mind so you don't think right, and make you do terrible things to avoid withdrawal."

"We all need help and fall short of the glory of God, though for most the enslavement is not as obvious, nor as socially devastating as it is with drug addiction. You can read about it in John 8.

*'Jesus replied, 'I tell you the truth, everyone who sins is a slave to sin. Now a slave has no permanent place in the family, but a son belongs to it forever. So if the Son sets you free, you will be*

*free indeed.'"*

"So, if I trust God, is He going to free me from hepatitis C?" asked Kyle.

"I don't know what miraculous answers to prayer God will perform in your future," I replied. "Like everyone else, you will have to trust God—believe that He loves you and pray continually with thanksgiving, with all types of prayer, on all occasions. I grant you that drug addiction comes with some awful consequences that will destroy your health, but that is the goal of evil—to steal, kill and destroy."

"I do want to be free of drugs, and fear they are destroying me. But as for the other stuff, I doubt a little lying, cheating, or pornography is going to harm anyone," offered Kyle.

"You are wrong there," I countered. "Other things may be more socially acceptable, with little risk of medical injury, but they still cause destruction in our lives. Things like pornography, TV and video games can be addicting. Given enough time they will rip apart families. Even a little lie left to fester will lead to the same end--loss of trust and ultimately damaged relationships."

"Come on, TV isn't going to kill you." Kyle laughed.

"Not anymore than taking hydrocodone for a broken arm, but given time and no boundaries it can draw you in. With TV it is not so much what it does to you, as what it keeps you from doing—participating in real life. You end up in a virtual reality that blinds you to the important things and sucks up your time. The true measure of life is in relationships, with family, friends and most importantly with God."

"Well, I'd trade drug addiction for video games or TV any day."

"And you would be no closer to being healed and really living. Trading addictions is a no-win. What good does it do you if you gain the whole world but forfeit your soul?"

Kyle thought for a moment and smiled, "This discussion

leads me to make a little joke. What's the difference between a drug addict and a doctor?"

"I give up, what?"

"The addict knows what death is." Kyle laughed at his own attempt at humor, then grew sullen again.

Sensing his growing melancholy I spoke, "This whole conversation is pretty depressing if not for one thing."

"What's that?" Kyle asked.

"Even though we are dead, God wants to help us. We just need to ask and seek Him. It reminds me of a verse I memorized as a child: *'So I say to you: Ask and it will be given to you; seek and you will find; knock and the door will be opened to you. For everyone who asks receives; he who seeks finds; and to him who knocks, the door will be opened.'" (Mark 8:36 NIV)*

"Do you really believe that?" Asked Kyle.

"Jesus gave it to us as a promise for those who seek His help. If you think about it, Jesus is the fulfillment of God's promise to help us. His resurrection becomes the proof that death and sin have been conquered. Those who seek Him will receive the power that raised Jesus from the dead unleashed in their own lives."

"I asked God for help once," said Kyle. "But nothing happened."

"Could our discussion right now be part of God's response to your prayer?" I offered.

"I was hoping for something a little more dramatic," said Kyle.

"You want instantaneous healing and no withdrawal?"

"Yeah, I have heard of others being healed like that, why not me?" questioned Kyle.

"I can't answer for others," I said searching for the right words to answer my own doubts. "It is through the trials and struggles of life that I am learning dependence upon God. The harder the struggle, the more I have to rely on Him. In the end I will see the 'why' of each difficulty, but for now I have to trust that God loves me and will carry me through to the finish."

A gentle peace settled upon me and brought to mind a verse I had read earlier:

*"Don't be afraid, for I am with you.*
*Don't be discouraged, for I am your God.*
*I will strengthen you and help you.*
*I will hold you up with my victorious right hand." Isaiah 41:10 NLT*

I silently gave thanks. Thank You Lord, for holding on to us through our worst times and making them into something for our good.

"Easy for you to say," Kyle broke into my thoughts. "Your life's not messed up like mine."

I looked at Kyle and prayed for God's wisdom and help. "Kyle, you look at me and see a white coat and a stethoscope, but underneath I struggle with failures, heartache and pride that cuts me off from God. I have regrets for my actions that have hurt my family. We both need forgiveness and the fullness of life found only in Jesus, and we both need a God who has the power to take our past and redeem it." I said putting my hand on Kyle's shoulder. "The twists and turns of life may be different, but one thing is clear—without God's love, we all would perish, but because of His love the ultimate triumph is assured."

"If only that were true," sighed Kyle.

"Here, take this prescription," I said, and proceeded to write out a promise for Kyle. "It is about the power of God's love to hold on to you."

Kyle read it out loud.

*"No, in all these things we are more than conquerors through him who loved us. For I am convinced that neither death nor life, neither angels nor demons, neither the present nor the future, nor any powers, neither height nor depth, nor anything*

*else in all creation, will be able to separate us from the love of God that is in Christ Jesus our Lord." Romans 8:37-39 NIV*

"I want you to pull it out and read it whenever you are feeling discouraged to remind yourself of the truth. It is something I have to do on a regular basis, so I won't spiral into self-recrimination. The old thought, 'I've messed up so much that God has given up on me,' is a lie."

"Thanks, I need to hear that," said Kyle.

CHAPTER 18

# God's Enduring Compassion

One thing about dealing with addictions—relapse is common. People have to learn recovery is one day at a time, yet lasts a lifetime. Through all this we can trust the Lord, and that His compassion is strong, undiminished, untarnished, bright, full, infinite in its reach, patient, and new every morning, regardless of what happened last night. Now, accepting all this to be true for yourself is another thing. How good is it that even in this God wants to help us.

I first met Allen for a work related injury. He tore up his shoulder when a wrench slipped while working on a truck engine. The post accident return-to-work and liability for medical expenses became complicated when the routine post-accident drug screen came back positive for cocaine.

"How can they not cover my medical treatment when my injury took place on the job," Allen protested?

"The company has claimed the cause of the accident to be your use of cocaine, and they are protesting to Workers Comp about having to cover this injury. Everything is on hold until Workers Comp investigates and makes a decision. In the meantime you need to stop using any drugs."

"Don't worry about that, I am not touching that stuff again," Allen declared.

They denied Allen's worker's compensation claim based on the positive drug test and he lost his job. Unfortunately, his use of cocaine did not stop, instead increased as a means of dealing with all his problems. One night, I got a call from the ER. Allen had been brought in following a car accident. He had driven off the road and hit a tree. Though the car was totaled, he had come through with only a few cuts and bruises.

As I finished sewing him up we talked.

"How did this happen? Did you fall asleep?" I inquired.

Allen stared at the ceiling with bloodshot eyes. "Yeah, something like that."

"What is the 'something' you're referring to?" I inquired. "Have you been using cocaine again?"

Allen stared at the ceiling and said nothing.

"Dr. Hufman," the ER nurse interrupted, "the police need to speak with you when you are finished."

"I'm done," I replied removing my gloves and looking up at the nurse. "Would you dress the wounds while I talk to the police?"

I stepped into the hall where the police were standing.

"We found this in the car." The officer held out a plastic bag with traces of white powder. "After you're done we are taking him in to be booked for possession of cocaine. We need to let you know that he'll be spending a few days in jail."

Returning to Allen, I told him what the police told me. "They can watch for infection at the jail, but I want to see you at my office in ten days to take out the sutures, and talk about your use of cocaine."

I did not see Allen again for about three months.

"Don't leave for lunch," my nurse warned me. "You have a last minute add-on—It's Allen." She rolled her eyes as she gave me his chart. "Oh, would you recheck his blood pressure? I got 165/100."

I entered the exam room to see a police officer standing beside the exam table where Allen sat. Allen's head and shoulders drooped in dejection, matching the orange jumpsuit and manacles. His hands nervously fingered the chain connecting the cuffs while he chewed on his lower lip.

The police officer spoke, "Allen was pulled over two nights ago for erratic driving, we found cocaine in the car. Having broken the conditions of his parole, the judge gave him six months at Deer Lodge (state prison). We're here to make sure he'll be okay for the six-hour trip. If you want, I can wait outside the door until you're done."

"Yes, thank you, I'll try not to be too long," I said as the officer stepped out and closed the door. I turned to face Allen. He looked horrid, and couldn't stop fidgeting on the table.

"Why didn't you come in like I instructed?" I said a little annoyed.

"I'm no good Doc," Allen blurted out. "I have nothing to live for…I have wasted every opportunity, burned every bridge, betrayed every friend, broken every promise, and destroyed my family. What's the use of going on?"

Allen's eyes were red and blood shot, he looked exhausted from detoxing in jail.

"What made you start again?" I asked looking for some clue as to how to proceed. I couldn't figure out how Allen had let himself relapse. What was he thinking?

"I don't know… I wish I did… After losing my job at the mill, I had to work two jobs to make ends meet. I needed something to keep me going." Allen said shaking his head. "I can't believe I did this again. I was clean until a week ago. My wife is going to leave with my kids over this. I might as well be dead." Allen began to shake.

Remembering the adage from medical training—make sure you find out what the patient is seeking before proceeding with medical care—I posed my next question. "So, what do you want from…?"

"You gotta give me something for my nerves," he said cutting me off. "I'm getting real drug sick."

"I can't do that," I said hoping jail time might wake him up. "You'll just have to ride this out in prison. It should ease over the next few days." I found it odd that Allen was looking at hard time for drug possession, and yet he wanted more drugs.

"You don't understand," pleaded Allen with his hands shaking. "I'm desperate. You got to give me something!"

"I will give you this," I said gathering my thoughts on what

I wanted to say. "Your life, your family's life, depends on whom you decide to trust in this hard time. You can continue to trust yourself, which is destroying your life, or you can put your trust in God and His mercy, which will restore life." I had little sympathy for Allen because I knew the terrible situation of his family.

"Why would God care?" Allen said looking surprised at my bluntness. "I don't even know if I believe in God. Besides, I'm the one who messed up."

"If God sent Jesus to die for you, don't you see that says something about how much He cares?" I felt a stab of guilt over my own lack of caring, but it ticked me off that Allen had done this to his wife and kids.

For a long moment Allen sat there. Then he spoke just above a whisper, "Jesus died for me? I never thought of it that way… Jesus has always been a swear word."

Now it was my turn to be surprised. I had no time to think when words poured out of my mouth.

"The prophets of the Old Testament made it clear that Jesus was the Messiah from God. The miracles Jesus performed testified of His authority. His death and resurrection proclaim triumph over all our sins and failures. Yes, I think you can say with conviction that Jesus is much more than a swear word, He is the lamb of God sent to rescue us." Whoa, where did that come from?

Allen stopped fidgeting and seemed to calm down. I worried he might take offense at my words, but plunged ahead anyway not able to stop. "When you get to Deer Lodge ask for a Bible and look up John 3:16-17. I believe God loves you and wants to pour out his mercy upon you."

I finished my exam and retook his blood pressure and pulse. Both had come down since my nurse had taken them. Looking again at Allen, I saw tears filling his eyes.

"Doc, I don't know how to do this… would you pray for me?"

Shocked at this change in Allen, I stumbled through a prayer. At the end Allen said, "Jesus, I want to give You my life—it's a mess."

As I watched Allen leave with the police officer, I stood there dumbfounded at what God had just done despite me.

Allen went to prison a changed man. He told his wife by phone and she couldn't believe it so she called me. We had a long talk which ended with her praying the same prayer as Allen. I then gave her some verses to share with Allen:

*"Because of the LORD's great love we are not consumed, for his compassions never fail.*
*They are new every morning; great is your faithfulness." Lamentations 3:22-23 NIV*

*"So from now on we regard no one from a worldly point of view. Though we once regarded Christ in this way, we do so no longer. Therefore, if anyone is in Christ, he is a new creation; the old has gone, the new has come!" 2 Corinthians 5:16-17 NIV*

*"I have come into the world as a light, so that no one who believes in me should stay in darkness." John 12:46 NIV*

Grace and peace came to Allen's family because of the LORD's great love.

SECTION 6

# Following Fear, or Following Jesus

So many choices in life to make.
How can you know which one to take?
Often it's fear that jerks the chain.
You fall in line to avoid the pain.
Where's the freedom, hardly a choice?
Oh, to follow a loving voice,
That knows each bend what lies in wait.
Has conquered all and changed ill fate.

by Stephen Hufman

How do you love a son, or a daughter, and watch them destroy themselves? When is helping enabling?

These questions hound everyone in the family of a person with addictions. Unfortunately, there is no easy answer. It is love's dilemma—when to act and when to hold back, when to hang on and when to let go. Even God suffers this pain in watching us choose to reject Him, but fortunately, His love has triumphed over death, and reaches out to embrace us… if we are willing.

*"O Jerusalem, Jerusalem, you who kill the prophets and stone those sent to you, how often I have longed to gather your children together, as a hen gathers her chicks under her wings, but you were not willing." Matthew 23:37 NIV*

CHAPTER 19

# Love's Dilemma

Kevin and Carla came to me asking for help with their son, Brian. In the spring of Brian's senior year, he started abusing hydrocodone.

"To live and love is to live in pain when there are drugs involved," said Kevin. "I feel like I have failed as a father..." Kevin stopped to clear his throat trying to gain control of his emotions.

"Please, forgive our tears," said Carla gently squeezing Kevin's hand. "This is such a nightmare for our family. We have been keeping this private for so long, it is crushing us."

Kevin was the pastor at the largest church in our small town, and I could see how this weighed heavily upon both of them.

"I may be a pastor," Kevin said, "but I don't have any answers when it comes to this stuff. I will say I've wondered if I should step down from the ministry. I mean, if I can't lead my own family how can I lead the church."

"Honey, we can't make all the decisions for our kids, and Brian is eighteen" interjected Carla. "You're a good Father and a fine pastor."

A long pause ensued in which I silently prayed for the Holy Spirit's strength.

With a halting voice Kevin unfolded their story.

~

Brian had been acting strange for about two months when Carla first brought up his odd behavior.

"Kevin, have you noticed a change in Brian?" Carla asked. "I'm worried that something is wrong."

"I think he's studying hard for finals," Kevin shrugged. "This being his senior year he has a lot on his mind."

"No, there is something else going on. Usually he charges through each day making the most of each moment. But lately, it's as if he doesn't care anymore."

"We used to call it senioritis. It can be intimidating going off to school on a basketball scholarship. Once he settles in and makes friends with his team mates—he'll be okay."

Kevin broke off the story to tell me that he felt a special pride in seeing his son excel at school and in sports.

"You know, after graduation, Brian would have been moving up to a bigger stage," Kevin said as tried not to lose composure. "We all relished the thought of watching him play ball at the university level. That was until this Spring when something began to overshadow Brian's usual energetic spirit. He became more petulant and withdrawn. Most uncharacteristic of all—he had stopped shooting hoops in the driveway. One Saturday evening he came home and went straight to his room avoiding everyone."

"Kevin, go talk to Brian and find out what's wrong," said Carla. "I'm worried that he is depressed or something."

"Aww, he's gonna be alright, Brian's going through growing pains of being eighteen and trying to find himself."

"Oh Kevin, please, go up and check on our son. It will make me feel a lot better," Carla insisted.

Kevin climbed the stairs thinking of all the times He had prayed for the family. Brian is the oldest of three children, next come Mary a 7$^{th}$ grader, and little Sandra in 3$^{rd}$ grade. Quickly he prayed for strength and the right words to say without sounding over-bearing.

Knock. Knock.

"Go away," came Brian's voice from behind the door.

"Brian, I want to talk with you."

Some movement occurred behind the door and it opened a crack.

"Yeah, what's-the-matter now?" Brian said in a dull monotone voice.

Kevin put his hand on the door knob and pushed to open it further. But Brian had blocked the door with his foot.

"Open the door, Brian. You may be eighteen and about to graduate but you are still my son living in our home."

The door opened, and Brian returned to his bed rolling with his pillow to face the wall.

"Brian, what is going on? Your mother and I are worried."

"I'm just tired, I have been up late the last few nights with homework."

"Look at me, Brian. It's more than a few nights of homework. You have been missing dinner, going out at strange hours, and plain rude to the rest of the family."

Brian turned and faced his father, but seemed to let his gaze drift like he was going to sleep.

"I'm pretty tired Dad, can we take this up tomorrow?"

"All right, we'll talk after church tomorrow."

"Dad, don't bother waking me for church, I'll just fall asleep in the pew… goodnight." Brian rolled back to the wall.

Kevin started to leave, but noticed a white tablet on the floor. Picking it up he asked, "What is this pill next to your bed?"

"I had a headache, so I burrowed some of Mom's medicine. Please, I just want to get some sleep." Brian said as he pulled his pillow over his ears. "You can leave now… and close the door."

Plagued by doubts Kevin returned to Carla.

"Well, that didn't go very well," he said answering Carla's look of worry. "Brian says he is too sleepy to talk now."

"That's it?" Carla said with deepening alarm. "My intuition says there is more going on than just being sleepy."

"Well, I did find this," showing Carla the pill. "Brian said he had borrowed some of your medicine for a headache."

"My medicine?" Carla said. "I don't have any medicine for headaches, other than Tylenol." Carla remembered something and took off to the bathroom. Soon she returned holding a pill bottle. "I have this old bottle of hydrocodone for pain from my knee surgery last year. I never needed them so there is still a full prescription."

"Maybe we should count them. It says there are sixty in this bottle." Kevin poured the pills onto a small plate and quickly counted them. "Sixty, so where did the tablet I found in Brian's room come from?"

"Wait a minute, something is not right. This pill doesn't match the others," Carla's voice began to tremble. "If he is telling the truth there should be less than sixty pills. Do you think he would…?"

"Don't go jumping to conclusions, Carla. There is probably a simple reason for the mix up. Maybe Brian meant to say he took some Tylenol." Fear made them both grab for any explanation other than what the evidence suggested.

Carla got the bottle of Tylenol from the medicine cabinet and compared the pills. "Look, none of these match."

"Carla, why don't you take the pills to the pharmacy Monday, and sort this out. Don't go and get all worked up about it. Brian is a good kid, I am sure we'll get it all straightened out." Secretly Kevin was just as scared as Carla, but didn't want to admit it. Looking back, Kevin realized that one of the sinister parts of drugs is they make the family stop talking with each other about their real feelings because everyone's afraid.

At that point, Kevin stopped his narration and gave Carla a hug. "I am sorry for being so unwilling to face the truth and trust your motherly intuition."

"I forgive you," said Carla. "To get through this we will both need to seek God's mercy at His throne of grace."

Kevin gave Carla another hug and returned to the story.

Brian stayed in his room the entire weekend, coming out

only to use the bathroom and get snacks from the kitchen. We both debated on what to do about Brian's behavior.

"Let's wait till Monday when you talk to the pharmacist about the pills," Kevin suggested. "I'm sure we will get it straightened out. If Brian claims he is not well enough to go to school, you can take him to see the doctor. Call me at the church if there's a problem."

Monday morning Brian got up; ate some toast with jam, and headed for the door.

"Brian, how is your headache?" asked Carla.

"Fine," said Brian as he side-stepped his mom to leave.

"Brian, don't you have a morning kiss for me?"

"Sure," Brian kissed the air next to Carla's cheek and shot out the door.

After cleaning up, Carla took the pills to the pharmacy.

Upon returning home she tried to figure all the possibilities, and called Kevin at church.

"Kevin," Carla's panicked voice came over the phone. "Brian stole my hydrocodone and replaced them with generic Tylenol. I'm certain Brian's behavior change is from using drugs!"

"Whoa, how did you come to that conclusion?" Kevin said, a little irritated with Carla's accusation.

At this point Kevin broke off telling me the story to point

Signs of possible drug use in adolescents:

Change in academic performance.
Missing school and other activities.
Defiance of authority.
Loss of interest in activities and hobbies.
Change in friends.
Isolation.
Acting secretive.
Lying.
Avoiding eye contact.
Isolation.

out how difficult it is to realize your son is using drugs. The slightest hint of that being possible tears you apart, and at first you refuse to even go there. But slowly, the pit in your stomach grows until you fall in. It is a dark dungeon of hurt and panic, mingled with blame toward everyone, especially yourself.

After a few moments, Kevin continued with the story, starting in at Carla's phone call.

"The pharmacist told me the pill you found in Brian's room is hydrocodone, the pills that should have been in the prescription bottle. The medicine in the bottle had been switched to acetaminophen to hide the theft. Kevin, what are we going to do?" Carla's voice grew tight with emotion.

Kevin fought with himself, barely able to stay calm. "It's not possible! We've raised him better than that. I can't believe Brian would be involved with drugs? We'll talk this over tonight when I get home. I am sure there is some logical explanation for this. You should call the school and see if they have noted any change in Brian's behavior."

"I already called them," Carla's voice trembled. "He is not at school today and missed two days last week."

"Let me wrap up a few things here, and I'll head straight home." Kevin's hands were shaking as he put the phone down. Not Brian… what could have happened to my son?

> In the US there are 7,800 new drug users a day, 54 percent of this group are under the age of 18. More than half of new illicit drug users begin with marijuana next most common entry drug is prescription pain medicine.

When Kevin arrived at home, Carla met me at the door with a worried look.

"What are we going to do?" Carla blurted out nearly crying.

"First, we will sit down with Brian and see what he has to say. Don't make this into more than it is. Every kid goes through an experimentation stage. We just need to do a little course correction with Brian, that's all."

"Kevin, it's bigger than that. I checked the petty cash pouch in the desk and it's empty. After that, I checked through the house to see if anything else is missing. I couldn't find some of my jewelry and Brian's hunting rifle is not in the locker."

Kevin collapsed into the chair his world spun out of control. Brian stealing and taking drugs? No, this couldn't be happening, it must be a dream. Lord, help!

Brian's car pulled into the driveway and he got out heading to the front door.

"We should talk to Brian before Mary and Sandra get home from school," Carla said.

The door opened. "Hey, Dad what are you doing home?" Brian said as he tried to pass by and go up to his room.

"Brian, your mom and I need to talk with you now."

"Okay." Brian said a little hesitantly. "But I'm having a little diarrhea can I at least drop off my school stuff and use the bathroom?"

"Be quick about it, your sisters will be home soon."

Brian raced up stairs to his room. They heard him shuffling around and walk into the bathroom.

After five minutes Kevin grew tired of waiting and climbed the stairs to knock on the bathroom door. "Brian, are you okay?"

"Sure, I'll be right down," came from behind the door.

After a few more minutes the toilet flushed and Brian stepped out. "Dad, I said I'd be right down, give me some space would you."

"Look at me, Brian. Something is not right. We need to talk now."

Brian's pupils were pinpoint, and he moved with a slight clumsiness. Upon reaching the living room, Brian plopped onto the sofa with his head on the armrest.

"Can we get this over with, I'm pretty sleepy? I was up late last night studying for a test today," Brian yawned and put his arm across his eyes.

"Don't lie to us," said Carla with a tinge of anger. "I checked with the high school and you were not there today."

"Well, I am eighteen and it is none of your business."

"You are not to talk to your mother like that. We are still your parents and something is wrong. Now why don't you start telling us what is going on?"

Brian shrugged and seemed to drift, he caught himself and started to talk, "I am really tired can we discuss this later?"

The kitchen door opened, and giggling announced the girls arrival.

"Mom, we're home. Can we have a snack?" Sandra's voice came from the kitchen.

Kevin stared at Brian wondering who had taken over his son? "We will have to talk later when you are not so sleepy. Go to your room. Dinner is at 6:30; you need to be there, and you had better be in school tomorrow."

Brian didn't respond, but got up and left for his room. Kevin looked at Carla.

"We need to take precautions until we figure this out. Don't leave any valuables lying about, lock them in the gun safe, I will change the padlock. In the morning, tell Brian that we will be checking his school attendance daily."

"Kevin, what are we going to do if Brian is using drugs? I should have flushed those pain pills long ago. What about Sandra and Mary I don't want them exposed to this."

"I don't know. We don't even know for sure if Brian is using. Maybe he has the flu or is depressed."

Carla stood up, "One of us should go check on him in case he really is sick."

"You go look after the girls and I'll go check on Brian." Kevin stood up and trudged up the stairs praying for wisdom but surrounded by fear. "How could this be happening to my family?" screamed through his mind.

CHAPTER 20

# No Light Ahead

Knock, knock.

"Brian, I need to talk with you," Kevin called through Brian's bedroom door. "Brian answer me or I am coming in."

No response. Turning the knob he pushed to open the door. But something prevented the door from moving more than a crack. Pushing harder, he looked in to see what blocked the door, and saw Brian's limp arm.

"Carla! Call 911! Brian's passed out on the floor!" With panic surging, Kevin pushed a little harder until the door opened enough that he could reach in and push Brian away from the door. Once inside, he tried to shake Brian awake... no response. Hands shaking he checked for a pulse... nothing but a limp arm. The fear mounted as he put his ear to Brian's chest... maybe a faint heart beat. "Carla, I'm starting CPR. Get help here quick!"

"Please Lord save my son," Kevin prayed over and over. Trying to mimic what he had seen on TV Kevin pulled Brian's jaw forward, pinched his nose, and blew two quick breaths and started pumping on his chest.

"Carla, is the ambulance coming!"

"What is happening? Lord almighty is he..." Carla cried out from the bedroom door.

"Carla, send the girls to the basement and go out to meet the ambulance. You can't help here," Kevin said not looking up from pumping on Brian's chest. After a 100 thrusts, he gave Brian two quick breaths and continued.

Finally the paramedics arrived. Near the dresser they saw a zip lock with white pill fragments, and quickly administered Narcan. Brian started to rouse as they loaded him in the ambulance.

At the hospital Brian regained consciousness, and lab tests confirmed he had suffered an opiate overdose. They watched him in the ER until they were sure he wouldn't rebound after the Narcan wore off, then released him to Kevin and Carla. The girls were with their grandparents for the night.

"Okay Brian, tell us what is going on," Kevin demanded. His hands still shook, so he griped the steering wheel and drove slowly through the dark deserted streets of town.

"Nothing's going on, I just took something to relax and forgot how many I had taken."

"Oh please, opiates are not for relaxing! Where did you get them?"

"Lots of kids pass them around at school."

"I think you need to be more specific," Kevin responded. "Tell us how long has this been going on. Where are you getting the narcotics and the money to pay for them?"

"Kevin, don't get angry," interjected Carla from the back seat. "Our boy almost died; he needs help. Brian, we need to know these things so we can help you."

"Don't worry Mom, I'll be fine. After tonight I won't be taking anymore. It's just not worth it." Brian stared out the window.

"That's good," said Carla.

"You still haven't answered my questions," Kevin said making the last turn toward home. Everything seemed so surreal like a bad dream, but Kevin knew there would be no waking up.

"Look, Dad, I'm sorry about tonight. I feel bad about overdosing, and I already told you, I am done with pills. So, you can drop the third degree."

"I want to believe you, but we have money and a gun missing, would you care to explain that?"

"I don't know anything about missing money, and the gun is mine. If you must know I went gopher hunting with a friend and left it at his house. Is every little thing going to be pinned on me because of one mistake?"

"Oh, Brian, we love you and are just worried about you. Your dad and I have been through a lot today, please understand we don't mean to accuse you…"

"Well, it sure feels like it," growled Brian.

Kevin pulled into the driveway and hit the garage door opener.

"I'm feeling a little rough after all this," said Brian. "If we're done with the interrogation I'd like to go to bed."

"Sure honey, I think a little sleep will do us all some good," said Carla trying to ease the tension.

Brian got out of the car, ducked under the rising garage door, and went straight to his room.

In anger, Kevin pulled into the garage shut the car off and turned to Carla. "He nearly killed himself with drugs today and you let him off the hook! He told us nothing except he had a little MISHAP. Why, we don't even know if he has more drugs stashed in his room." Laying his head on the steering wheel, Kevin fought to keep his emotions in check.

"Brian is our son, not some criminal," protested Carla.

"I know he's our son, I just don't know how much to trust what he says."

The overhead garage door light clicked off plunging them into an inky gloom.

"Honestly I'm torn. I want to believe Brian, I just don't know what to believe," said Carla, her tears hidden by the darkness.

After wrestling with his thoughts, Kevin muttered, "Maybe we should pray for help."

Kevin stopped the story and looked at me with tears in his eyes. "That was the lowest point in my life… in our lives." Kevin put his arm around Carla before going on. "I was angry, afraid and stood at a crossroad. I wanted to yell at Carla and go in the house and grab Brian to pound some sense into him. But there, in the darkness, a verse came to mind:

> *"Fear not, for I have redeemed you; I have summoned you by name; you are mine. When you pass through the waters, I will be with you; and when you pass through the rivers, they will not sweep over you. When you walk through the fire, you will not be burned; the flames will not set you ablaze. For I am the Lord, your God, the Holy One of Israel, your Savior." Isaiah 43:1-3*

I had to make a choice at that moment between doing something rash, or bowing before Jesus and trusting Him. All I can say is this may not be over, but Jesus goes with me, and that is what I need."

> Healthy families have trust in each other. But with addictions trust is destroyed, wreaking havoc on relationships by coloring every interaction with suspicion. Some family members will cope by distancing themselves and avoidance. Others will be caught up in the mess and limp along in codependency. Their love tries to maintain some kind of relationship regardless of the consequences. Codependent relationships usually end up enabling the addictive behavior to continue. This is love's dilemma: when does love cease to be love and becomes something less?

After a brief pause, Kevin continued.

Over the next few days, Brian seemed to be more like his old self. At least that is what Carla and Kevin told themselves.

"How is school going?" asked Carla each morning when Brian entered the kitchen.

Brian usually responded with "fine," grabbed some toast or

a Pop-Tart and left.

In the evening it would be more of the same: no conversation, just take some food and disappear.

"I've had enough of this," Kevin said to Carla after drying the evening dishes. "If Brian wants to eat, he can sit at the kitchen table and be sociable."

"Oh Kevin," responded Carla. "The boy is only eighteen after all. Go easy on him, it's only been one week since his accident."

"Accident! He almost kills himself and we still know nothing. We need to find out what's going on, not make excuses for him."

On impulse Kevin bounded up the stairs and knocked on Brian's door. "Brian, come on out...we need to talk."

"Dad, can it wait? I'm right in the middle of writing a paper for English Lit."

"It won't take long. We just need to set up some rules around here."

"Okay, I'll be down as soon as I finish this paragraph."

Kevin went downstairs determined to lay down some rules. After closing the door to the TV room where the girls were watching videos, he sat down in his easy chair across from the couch, where Carla sat holding tightly to her handkerchief.

"I am worried if we push too hard he'll leave. Then what will we do?" Carla said just above a whisper.

"So how do you know he is not still using drugs? You agree we can't have that around the girls, don't you?"

"I'm his mother, I think I know him well enough to tell if he is hiding something."

"Yeah, well why didn't you notice something was wrong before he overdosed?" Kevin's words hurt Carla. "Sorry, I didn't mean to blame you like that." The truth is it was my denial that had blinded us to the signs of trouble.

"I love Brian," Carla dabbed her eyes with her handkerchief. "I think he just needs a little time right now."

"Well, I think we need to set some house rules."

"And if Brian doesn't agree to them, what are you going to do?"

"He..." Kevin stopped upon hearing Brian open his bedroom door.

Brian shuffled down the stairs and plopped on the couch, "Okay, let's get it over with. What do we need to talk about?" Brian said with sarcasm.

Both Carla and Kevin stared at Brian trying to discern any hint of narcotics.

"You both are acting weird. I am going back upstairs," said Brian.

"Umm... not so fast son, we need rules about how we are going to act in this house... starting with treating each other with courtesy, and civility."

"Is that all? You had me come down here for that?"

"No," Carla broke in. "We want to know that you are all done with drugs."

"I already told you I'm not taking any more pills. What do you want me to do, take a lie detector test?"

"No, but a urine drug screen would go a long way to reassure us." Kevin said.

"Oh, so my word is not good enough any more?" Brian's voice took on a hard edge.

Carla quickly recovered from the surprise of Kevin's request, "Brian darling, we trust you. It's just your father is worried about you. You can understand that, can't you?"

"So what happens if I say no?" Brian countered.

"Refusing will signal to me that you are still using drugs," Kevin shot back.

"Then what, Dad?" Brian chided.

"Your mom and I don't want you in the house around your sisters if you're using drugs."

"So you are going to throw me out because you don't trust me. What happened to love that always protects, always trusts, always hopes, always perseveres." Brian got up looked at his mom and said, "One mistake and you want to kick me in the gutter what kind of love is that?" With that he turned and went back to his room.

Carla looked at Kevin in shock. "You're going to throw our son out on the street because he won't get a drug screen? That would cause worse problems. You want Brian finding refuge in some drug house? At least here we can help if he is still using. If he had overdosed on the street, he might be dead!"

> Not every medical clinic is set up to do urine drug screens. In the clinics that do drug screens they will require that the report go to a legally responsible entity (doctor, lawyer, court or company in case of work place screening). The report will not be open to the family for a person eighteen or older. Therefore just dropping by to ask for a test is not going to happen. The best way is to go through an addiction specialist or have your primary care provider order the test. Even then the results go to the patient (if over 18) not the parents. Other considerations in this process: 1. Being assured that the patient does not game the system (the Internet is full of ways to pass urine drug screens). 2. Not all drugs of abuse are tested with office urine drug screens. 3. How are the results going to be used, will there be legal ramifications such as child custody disputes, or parole violation.

"Honestly, I don't know what's right? I don't even know what love means. I love Brian, but I can't sit here and do nothing."

The next five weeks were difficult with only a thin veneer of normalcy, until one night Brian announced he had dropped out of school to work full time.

"What!" Kevin exploded. "If you want to stay in this house, then you'll stay in school. Graduation is only a few weeks away. What are you thinking?"

"Dad, whether or not you agree, it's done. I am eighteen and it is my decision. If you want to kick me out that's your decision I can stay with my friends till I find my own place."

"Brian, why are you doing this?" Carla cried. "What is wrong? This is not like you."

"I'm going out," said Brian. "I think you and Dad need to talk. I'll be back late so don't wait up. We can talk more tomorrow."

"Brian, you're using drugs, aren't you?" Kevin shouted following Brian to his car.

"Careful Dad, the neighbors may be listening." Brian got in his car and left.

Bewildered, Kevin closed the front door. Carla sobbed on the couch.

"Daddy, where is Brian going?" came Mary's voice from the top of the stairs.

"It's okay darling, you go back to bed." Kevin felt the sting of misleading his daughter, aghast at how drugs affected the entire family.

> Drugs make people into liars and cheats, because they are trying to hide the truth from themselves and people around them. Love rejoices with the truth which is fundamental to good relationships for it builds trust. A hard question for families is where does love stop and enabling begin? A clue is that love always seeks to restore a right relationship, and won't allow anything less. Where enabling will settle for any relationship, even one that is built on a lie, or filled with resentment.

"Carla, come into the kitchen," said Kevin. "We need to

pray. I'm barely holding it together."

"Me too," responded Carla.

They held each other's hand at the table and Kevin began, "Lord, from the time of his birth we have prayed for Brian. Right now, we don't know what to say, but our sorrow and fear are overwhelming. Please, help us. Show us what to do. Watch over Brian and protect him from evil, and bring him home safe. Amen."

"Do you think he's using drugs again?" Carla asked.

"I don't think he ever stopped," Kevin replied.

"What are we going to do? I feel so helpless."

"First, we'll check Brian's room, the bathroom, and any place he might have used to stash drugs. If we find any evidence of drugs, we can confront him when he gets home and get him into rehab."

The search produced nothing conclusive. Hearing Brian's car pull up, they quickly put things back closed drawers, and were at the top of the stairs when Brian entered the front door.

"Caught you going through my stuff didn't I?" Defiance dripped from Brian's voice. "This place has turned into a prison." Brian turned around and slammed the door as he left.

"Kevin, go bring him back!" sobbed Carla.

"How do I do that? He is eighteen, I can't kidnap him. He would resent and rebel against us more than he does now."

"Couldn't we accept him back drugs and all? Then we could at least monitor how he is doing, and talk him into drug treatment," Carla sobbed.

~

Love's dilemma is deciding when loving someone means letting them go. You can do everything and have all wisdom, yet if you force your will upon the one loved, it ceases to be love and becomes enslavement for both sides.

*"Jesus continued: 'There was a man who had two sons. The younger one said to his father, 'Father, give me my share of the estate.' So he divided his property between them. Not long after that, the younger son got together all he had, set off for a distant country and there squandered his wealth in wild living." Luke 15:11-13 NIV*

Jesus knows fully the pain of watching your child wander into harm's way.

*"As He approached Jerusalem and saw the city He wept over it..." Luke 19:41 NIV*

Therefore, we can with great assurance approach the throne of grace.

*"So then, since we have a great High Priest who has entered heaven, Jesus the Son of God, let us hold firmly to what we believe. This High Priest of ours understands our weaknesses, for he faced all of the same testings we do, yet he did not sin. So let us come boldly to the throne of our gracious God. There we will receive his mercy, and we will find grace to help us when we need it most." Hebrews 4:14-16 NIV*

CHAPTER 21

# Lies, Fear and Humility

Several weeks passed with the only contact from Brian coming in the form of showing up late at night asking for money or to get some of his clothes. At first they acquiesced giving in to his demands, thinking at least he's alive and doing okay. But then it became obvious that everything fueled Brian's drug use. They finally agreed to not give Brian any more money, food, or clothes. Also, they were not going to let Brian in the house because he would steal things, plus they didn't want the girls seeing their brother like this.

On Brian's next visit Kevin met him at the door to lay out the rules and block him from coming in.

"You can't come in this house anymore unless you are involved in rehab."

"Does Mom agree with you?"

"We have talked this over and she is in the kitchen ready to call the police if you try to force your way in."

"Mom," Brian called out. "I just need a hundred bucks and a place to stay. Don't force me to go out on the street."

"That's your choice Son, but we will no longer be dragged into your drug use," Kevin said with all the strength he could muster. "There is no way I'm giving you money to kill yourself. We love you too much to go along with your self-destruction."

"Okay, maybe I do have a drug problem, but help me out tonight and in the morning I'll start whatever program you want, I promise." Brian seemed to grow a little agitated.

"Kevin, why not let him stay here tonight, so we can start early at getting Brian into drug rehab." Carla spoke from the hallway.

"Carla! We agreed Brian can't stay here if he is still using drugs. For the sake of our family, we can't back down on this."

"Just for tonight," Carla pleaded. "If something were to happen tonight, I could never forgive myself."

"Dad, listen to Mom. I'll even sleep on the couch."

"Carla, we have to stick together on this." Kevin felt betrayed and angry at the whole situation.

"At least let me use the bathroom," said Brian. "I'll use the one off the laundry room so I won't contaminate your precious home."

Stepping aside, Kevin reluctantly let Brian pass. Then turning to Carla whispered, "Why didn't you back me up? I thought we had settled this plan between us?"

"I know, but I worry about Brian being out there and that something terrible will happen."

"Well, something terrible has happened, drugs have taken control of our son!"

"He said he'll go to rehab in the morning," pleaded Carla. "I think this is our chance to help him get treatment."

"Okay, but next time if we agree to a plan you have to back me up on it."

They heard the toilet flush Brian came out. Carla went over to Brian and gave him a big hug. "You can stay tonight but then tomorrow you go to drug rehab."

"Thanks Mom, I knew I could count on you," said Brian.

"Whew, you need a shower. I'll get you some clean clothes from upstairs while you clean up," she said hurrying off.

Kevin stood there unsure of what to say or do, feeling guilty for harboring doubts about his own son.

Brian went back to the bathroom, tossed his clothes on the laundry room floor, and took a hot shower. When he came out Carla had the couch all ready.

Kevin noticed a little wobble in Brian as he walked into the kitchen.

"Brian, did you just take drugs?" he inquired.

"Dad, you didn't want me getting the shakes tonight did you? I wouldn't have gotten any sleep. Besides, I don't want my family seeing me like that."

"Carla, come in here please."

"I have Brian's bed all made," she said walking into the kitchen.

"Brian just took some drugs," Kevin announced clenching his hand trying to maintain control.

Brian sat down and began to drift.

"Oh Brian, why?" said Carla.

"Mom, you and Dad just don't understand, I get real sick without them."

"Brian, we understand, but this has been difficult on all of us," Carla said.

"Mom... I need a hundred bucks." Brian said without lifting his head.

"That's the last thing you need," Kevin exclaimed.

"No, you don't realize, I took the pills already and told them you would give me the money to pay them back. If I don't get it for them tonight, they'll come looking for me. They know I'm here and are waiting down the block for me now."

"You mean you put your family in danger for drugs!" Kevin rose gripping the table with both hands. "I'll call the police if they come here."

"Dad, it doesn't work that way. If I don't get them the money they'll kill me."

"Kevin, give him the money!" cried Carla.

"Mom, what's happening?" Sandra stood at the hall door in her pajamas, rubbing her eyes.

"Carla you get Sandra back to bed and I'll take care of this."

When Carla had left with Sandra, Kevin turned to face Brian. "I wish I could beat some sense into you. Why are you doing this to us, and your sisters?"

"I don't know. I never thought it would be like this," said Brian.

"This is not the real you. These drugs make you act crazy… here take the money and tell those punks to stay clear… Brian, listen to me, you need to kick these drugs. They're killing you."

Brian stuffed the cash in his pocket and left.

"Where is Brian?" Carla asked upon returning from taking Sandra back to bed.

"I gave him the money to pay off his drug debts, and he left."

"Is he coming back? What are we going to do?"

"Go to bed, I'll wait up for Brian, though I am not sure he's coming back. This may have all been a charade to get money and a shower. I don't know what to believe anymore."

"I can't sleep not knowing if Brian is safe," said Carla. "Go out and find him and bring him back."

"You want me to tackle him and throw him in the car? Then what? Lock him in his room until morning and take him kicking and screaming to drug rehab. How long do you think that will last?"

"Well, at least it is something," said Carla.

"What about the drug pushers? It could make it more dangerous than it already is. I don't want them coming around here… think of Mary and Sandra!"

"You're right," admitted Carla. "I just find it hard to think straight when I picture Brian in some alley doing drugs. If I could just talk some sense into him."

"I don't think it would get very far. When Brian is using drugs it is like he is not there. Until Brian decides he wants to be clean, there is not much we can do except pray," Kevin said. Looking out the window he wondered if he would see Brian again, or even get through this alive.

"What if he comes back and needs more money, or needs clean clothes...or food?" asked Carla.

"Good point. We need to make a plan of how we will interact with Brian. One that we both promise to stick to this time." Kevin felt annoyed that Carla had caved in to Brian's manipulation.

"Kevin, I'm afraid for Brian. What happens if he dies… I

could never forgive myself."

Kevin looked at his wife. "If he dies, would you be able to forgive me?"

"Honestly, I don't know." Carla looked down into her lap trying to hide her apprehension. "I am so hurt and confused by all this… let's not talk about death, I don't want to go there."

"These drugs are destroying our relationship with Brian. I think it will make everything a lot worse if we let it destroy our love for each other. We have to come together on this or we will fall apart. Let us right now commit to each other and to seeking God's wisdom each day."

"And how do you propose we do that?" asked Carla.

"We can talk and pray together daily and be honest about our feelings," Kevin said. "Then we can seek help about what to do from people who are knowledgeable about this. People we both trust to give us wise godly advice."

"The pastor needs counseling?" asked Carla. "Are you willing to listen?"

Kevin knew what Carla meant—he had a fear of not being in control. As the leader, he was supposed to have all the answers, but Brian's addiction went way beyond his understanding. After a hard swallow he said, "Yes, I hope so."

"And what about Brian in the meantime?" Carla prodded.

"Whatever happens, I want you to know I love you, and I promise to do everything I can to keep Brian from killing himself, as long as it doesn't jeopardize the rest of the family."

"I'm just so worried," said Carla.

"Me too," Kevin lamented. "We just need to keep our focus on Jesus. He loves us, and I know He loves Brian. I read this verse this morning, and it's stuck in my mind.

*'For we were so utterly, unbearably crushed that we despaired of life itself. Why, we felt that we had received the sentence of death; but that was to make us rely not on ourselves but on God who raises the dead…'" 2 Corinthians 1:9 NIV*

Kevin interrupted telling me the story to make sure I understood the full measure of despair he and Carla felt.

"Words cannot express how dark and lonely this has been for Carla and me, but through it we are learning to rely upon God in ways we never imagined. I must say that sharing this with you is very difficult because we are ashamed of our failings as parents, and as leaders in Christ's church. But I trust that you will keep us in your prayers as we share this burden with you."

"Yes, I promise. I'm praying for God's intervention and that He strengthen you for all that lies ahead." I said with my heart breaking for this family.

Kevin told me that they had sought counseling in another town and had developed a strategy for dealing with Brian. Together they pledged not to deviate from the plan unless they both agreed to the change and had discussed it with their counselor. My role would be for support and prayer.

The first item they had agreed to institute was to stop all monetary support for Brian unless he was clean and taking part in a recovery program. They canceled their credit cards, and got new ones to insure Brian could not tap into their credit. Then they took Brian off their phone plan. Carla worried that if Brian had an emergency, he wouldn't be able to call for help. But after praying and talking about it, Kevin and Carla realized that Brian used his phone to get drugs, and that would definitely kill him—something they wanted no part of.

One area they didn't expect being so difficult and troubling came from within—fear. At every turn it popped out: "What if Brian gets ill? What if we make a mistake? What if we haven't done enough? What if God doesn't save Brian?"

"I know the Bible says that perfect love casts out fear," said Kevin. "I just never realized fear would keep trying to return. To my dismay, I have to constantly refocus on Jesus. You'd think as a pastor I would have this covered, but every day I have to work at it anew."

He paused in deep thought, struggling whether to go on.

"I don't expect you to fully understand what Carla and I have been going through," said Kevin. "I certainly did not until now. But I would cherish your prayers and quiet support."

I nodded.

Kevin then went on with his family's story.

CHAPTER 22

# The End of the Beginning

One night, Carla heard movement downstairs.

"Kevin, wake up! Someone is in the house! Did you lock the door when you came to bed?"

"Huh, what's happening?" Kevin said coming out of a deep sleep.

"Listen, I think I heard something moving. Look out the window, and see if you can see anything," whispered Carla.

"There is a car parked in front. It looks like Brian's. Stay here, and I'll go down and see. If you hear a commotion call the police."

He grabbed his robe and crept downstairs. Fear bounded through every part of his body.

Kevin stopped the story briefly to interject his own reflection on this episode. "You would think a man of faith would pray the whole way, but I'm sorry to say I was so scared it didn't even cross my mind. I cherish the verse Romans 8:26 in a whole new way. 'In the same way, the Spirit helps us in our weakness. We do not know what we ought to pray for, but the Spirit himself intercedes for us with groans that words cannot express.' I may not have been all I should as Christ's disciple, but Jesus was there with me." Kevin smiled, "Through all this I have grown in my dependence on God's grace. I have experienced firsthand a love greater than all my fears. A precious flow beyond what I can convey."

After a moment of quiet reflection, Kevin went on with the story.

"In the darkness of the living room Kevin saw a lone figure he recognized as Brian stuffing things into a sack."

"Brian! What are you doing?" he said flipping on the lights.

Brian jumped, then turned to face his father. "I have come back to get my stuff. Is that okay with you?"

"I don't believe you. You are stealing to get more drugs." Kevin could hear Carla coming down the stairs behind him.

"Stealing? I am just getting my stuff. Let me have it, and I'll get out of YOUR house, if that's what you think."

"Brian, are you okay?" Carla said as she stepped forward.

"Brian, you have to leave unless you're wanting to go to rehab. So empty the sack and get out," said Kevin.

"Some parents you turned out to be. You cancel my phone and credit card. What do you expect of me—bring you candy and flowers?"

"Brian, we love you," said Carla. "Can't you see we are only trying to do what is best for..."

"If you love me, then help me. I am living in my car under the viaduct. Is that what you want?" Brian's anger flared.

"Brian, you must leave now!" Kevin said as Carla gripped his arm. He could feel her quietly sobbing. "It's obvious you are still using drugs, but we still love you and won't settle for anything less than the fullness of Christ in you. So know this—we are ready to help when you are ready to receive it. Only it is by our rules, not yours."

Brian left mumbling, "If I die out there, you both are to blame."

Carla started to follow Brian, but Kevin held her back. "Remember, our plan. Let him go."

"But what if..."

"He dies?" Kevin finished Carla's thought, then added. "I don't know, but I do know if we keep dwelling on 'what ifs' we will second-guess ourselves into a straight jacket. We can't let ourselves be manipulated by the drugs Brian is using. We have to trust God."

Carla continued to fight her fears. "What was that verse you always quote from James? "*But when he asks, he must believe and not doubt, because he who doubts is like a wave of the sea, blown and tossed by the wind.*" Well,… I can't do it."

Kevin searched for words to encourage Carla, but his own fears pushed aside every other thought. He realized now how self-righteous he had sounded throwing around James 1:6. From deep within came a heart-felt prayer: Lord, help!

"God is asking me for something I can't produce," Carla said tears streaming down her cheeks. "I am a mother worried for her son, how do I get past that?"

"I have to admit, right now, I'm poor at the faith part too."

"Poor at faith,… hmm." Carla turned it over in her mind, "'*Blessed are the poor in spirit, for theirs is the kingdom of heaven.*' Do you think this verse from the Beatitudes is referring to us?"

"Well, maybe when you know you're spiritually poor, that's the time to ask God for what you don't have," Kevin suggested.

"You think God will help us with the faith we're missing?"

"How about the man with the epileptic son? He told Jesus '*I do believe, help me overcome my unbelief,*' and Jesus helped him."

"Yeah, but every few minutes my fear for Brian pops up and I begin to lose it," Carla sighed. "Maybe that's the way it is supposed to be? So that way we pray without ceasing, relying on God and not ourselves. Even when we are faithless, He is faithful."

Kevin stopped the story and gave Carla a hug in an effort to regain composure. Finally he spoke. "I have come to realize that there comes a time where the valley of the shadow of death is deeper and darker than I ever thought possible. To be honest, we constantly battle with blaming ourselves and blaming each other."

"Pray for us," said Carla. "For each day we face the choice between trusting God or yielding to fear and panic. It's the hardest lesson I've ever had to learn and keep learning—to rely on Jesus for everything, even faith. I keep thinking about how the disciples felt when Jesus asked them if they wanted to leave.

> *'You do not want to leave too, do you?" Jesus asked the Twelve. Simon Peter answered him, "Lord, to whom shall we go? You have the words of eternal life. We believe and know that you are the Holy One of God.' John 6:67-69 NIV*

"I bet they were scared like me, but had nowhere they could go," Carla said with a weak smile.

A week later, Brian called to let his parents know he would be going to LA with a friend. The news crushed Carla and Kevin.

"I can't talk for long. My friend has limited minutes on this phone," said Brian.

"But how will we contact you? How will we know you are safe?" Carla cried.

"I guess you should have thought of that before you cut me off," Brian replied, then hung up.

Kevin spoke with tears welling up in his eyes. "I thought things couldn't get any worse. Surely, after all our prayers... but Brian leaving for LA felt like a free-fall into hopelessness."

For the next six months everyone prayed. Carla told me of jumping every time the phone rang hoping it would be Brian dreading it would be some ER informing them of Brian's death. Each step in their terrible valley of death became just as frightening as the last, each prayer became a labor of effort not to give up. Kevin began calling their stumbling journey of faith "Yea steps," a weak attempt at humor based on the Twenty-Third Psalm.

> *"Yea, though I walk through the valley of the shadow of death, I will fear no evil; for thou art with me." Psalm 23:4 NIV*

Carla tolerated the joke knowing it helped Kevin cope.

Soon she added her own little twist to give herself some semblance of cheer—"Yay, for thou art with me." Through it all they both became more dependent on each other and upon God, often reminding each other: "Yea, for thou art with me." But they prayed this asking God to be there for Brian, as well as themselves.

One day, Carla answered the phone and squealed with joy recognizing Brian's voice.

"Mom, I am calling to let you know I am all right. I love you and am sorry for all the anguish I have caused."

"Where are you? Can we do anything to help? When can we see you?"

"Mom, slow down. I am in the Union Rescue Mission in LA. They have a drug rehab program. I have been clean now for thirty days, but still have a long way to go."

"Well, we'll fly down and see you. Do you need anything?" Carla could hardly contain her joy.

"Mom, I can't have visitors just yet. Only those in the rehab program can come on the floor and I'm not far enough along in treatment to have freedom to go outside. So you and Dad keep praying and I will talk to you again. There is one thing…"

"Yes, what is it?" Carla urged Brian to keep talking.

"I have contracted hepatitis C, and may need help to pay for medicine."

"Of course, let us know where and how much," responded Carla. "Do you need anything else; are you seeing a good doctor?"

"Mom, I am in good hands. I will call you again in a week. Tell Dad…" Brian started to tear up, "Tell Dad I'm sorry. I know I have caused you both a lot of distress, and I can't even promise that it is over. What I can tell you is God has given me a promise I want to share with you: 'Yea, though I walk through the valley of the shadow of death, I will fear no evil; for thou art with me; Thy rod and thy staff, they comfort me.' I know God is with me and that makes all the difference. I also know

God is with you, and that knowledge gives me assurance that my struggle with drug addiction hasn't caused you irreparable damage. Keep praying for me—I am praying for you."

Soon after Kevin and Carla with Mary and Sandra moved to LA to be closer to Brian. I continue to pray for them and know someday I will praise God for His enduring love that even covers "love's dilemma."

SECTION 7

# Practical Steps to Recovery

*"Where there is no vision, the people are unrestrained, but happy is he who keeps the law." Proverbs 29:18 NIV*

The following section lays out practical guidelines you can initiate to begin your own recovery program. The goal is to restore your vision of the true blessings of life and get yourself on a path out of addiction's trap.

CHAPTER 23

# Where to Begin?

A patient's first step to recovery has two parts: The first part is to become conscious of his/her desperate situation. The second is the desire to change in a direction that brings life. As the verse from Proverbs 29 infers—where there is no vision (true understanding), the person will not want to seek recovery. Getting past denial and to a point of desiring change can be difficult for those caught up in addictions. I hope that through the stories in this book, the reader will see his or her own desperate need and pursue the fullness of God's love and help. For those trying to help someone in the process of recovery, a clear understanding of their own weaknesses and boundaries is paramount. Otherwise, they may become part of the problem

*"What shall we conclude then? Are we any better? Not at all! We have already made the charge that Jews and Gentiles alike are all under sin." Romans 3:9 NIV*

Real help must come with compassion and humility clear of any legalistic hypocrisy. For all involved to get where God wants you will require God's help.

*"'Not by might nor by power, but by my Spirit,' says the Lord Almighty." Zechariah 4:6 NIV*

Humility is the critical component of any recovery, for with it the power of the Kingdom of Heaven is unleashed.

*"God blesses those who are poor and realize their need for him, for the Kingdom of Heaven is theirs." Matthew 5:3 NLT*

Treatment starts with stripping away all the denials and rationalizations that are used for coping with addiction. But with this removal of defense mechanisms they need to be given a lifeline of hope, or the sorrow can become unbearable. Regrettably, some overdoses are intentional from people seeing the awful truth of their addiction but having no hope—"What's the use?" or "I don't want to live like this anymore." Therefore, those helping must also put forth the love and hope that God offers to all in Jesus (His name means 'God saves'). A support group infused with God's love is important throughout recovery (usually a 12-step group). The group will not only give help over the rough patches of rehabilitation but also prevent the person from falling back into old habits by working through and applying the 12-steps. As people help each other, they help themselves. As people learn to love each other, they learn to love themselves.

"There is no pit so deep, that God's love is not deeper still."
Corrie ten Boom

Unfortunately, if the person trapped in addictions remains in denial and doesn't believe that their situation is desperate, then they will find it difficult to wholeheartedly commit to recovery. A strong desire to change is essential to persevering through all the hard work of recovery. This initial step of recognizing their desperate need for God's help and strength cannot be bypassed and often needs to be repeated because addictions do not easily release their grip. When the desperation of the situation starts to be muddled by rationalizations, then the self-sacrifice necessary for change seems more optional than absolutely necessary. That's the start of drifting into "my way" instead of "God, help me."

Typical rationalizations:

- "I've lost everything already. This is the only thing keeping me going."
- "Maybe I am not meant to be clean and sober."
- "I am tired and need a break to relax and gather my strength."
- "I am much more pleasant to be around when I've taken something."
- "Addictions run in my family; you can't fight against genetics."
- "I am under a lot of stress right now…"
- "If you were married to my spouse, you'd drink too."
- "No one can help me; so, I am self-medicating."

> Over 60% of people who receive treatment for substance abuse will relapse within the first year.

Interventions are used to convince the addicted person that they have a serious problem and they need help. By having a group of close friends and family confront the person, it is easier to refute the lies, and avoid being manipulated. It is important the group acts out of love, and constantly communicates their love to the person struggling with addictions. If the group strays from surrounding the person in love, then the subject of the intervention will get defensive and discount everything said. Without love the intervention becomes nothing but a "clanging cymbal." (1 Corinthians 13:1)

For family members involved in an intervention, acknowledgement needs to be made that they may be part of the problem. But this realization should not subvert the goal of the intervention, which is getting the addicted person to realize their desperate need for sobriety. The family members will have to work on their own codependency for complete healing. Family relationships often become warped by addictions, and if not dealt with, this family dysfunction can become an impediment to recovery (there are groups for codependents and excellent resources about codependency). For this reason, the support group and mentor should not be immediate family.

After the addicted person takes responsibility and admits he or she has an addiction, then they must commit to working on recovery. This commitment includes the family. Some members of the family may not be interested in helping because they have to attend to their own needs. That should not serve as a roadblock for making a commitment to recovery, for the real success depends on one's reliance on God, not circumstances of one's life or family.

One of the hardest parts of recovery is making an honest and sincere commitment. It is difficult to be honest because addictions make those under its control lie and cheat, especially to oneself. I guarantee the addicted person has promised themselves more than once they would quit, yet each time the promise evaporates under the pressure of withdrawal. So do not let the commitment to recovery be about promising to stay clean, instead it needs to be a commitment to daily partake in the grace of God. To seek His help in all things, even when you have failed for the hundredth time.

*"Forgetting the past and looking forward to what lies ahead, I press on to reach the end of the race and receive the heavenly prize for which God, through Christ Jesus, is calling us." Philippians 3:13-14 NLT*

It is similar for friends and family, they will need to daily seek God's strength, direction and grace.

*"I waited patiently for the Lord to help me,*
*and he turned to me and heard my cry.*
*He lifted me out of the pit of despair,*
*out of the mud and the mire.*
*He set my feet on solid ground*
*and steadied me as I walked along.*
*He has given me a new song to sing,*
*a hymn of praise to our God." Psalm 40:1-3 NLT*

Then there is the problem of pride—the cement in the wall of denial and many other obstacles in life.

*"Before his downfall a man's heart is proud, but humility comes before honor." Proverbs 18:12 NIV*

Pride, humility, and shame need to be understood and addressed by everyone involved with addictions. These are critical items in everyone's life, and especially so in addiction treatment.

For the person caught up in addictions, pride is the main thing that binds them from even beginning on the road to recovery (it's called denial). "I don't have a problem," they think, but it is pride talking. Unless humility comes to the rescue, the addict will remain trapped by drugs. Later on in recovery, pride will cause the person to slip back into relapse with thoughts like: "I can handle this," or "I'm can make my own rules now." The only way to crush pride is with humility before God: "Forgive me and help me to follow you," and "Not my way, O Lord, but Thy will be done."

Some doctors claim shame is the culprit that keeps people from seeking help. Thus they attempt to get rid of shame by calling addictions a disease. That approach unfortunately negates the important role of shame, namely to stir a hunger for something better, and provide a strong push to ask God for forgiveness. Once forgiven, the patient will go on to seek help from Jesus to become all God wants them to be. The shame they once experienced now becomes a prime reason for not wanting to return into the muck and mire of addictions.

Pride can also affect the family of the addicted person. They can be in denial about their family member's addiction, or even worse, try to force their own ideas of what to do upon the patient, making the problem more intransigent. Humility encourages family discussion by being transparent and open. It allows room to seek help, and maintains family relationships, all of which are important in any recovery. Any shame the family feels should be discussed and become a reason for supporting each other. Shame left in the shadows often becomes a source for misunderstanding that can drive a family apart.

> *"Blessed are those who hunger and thirst for righteousness, for they will be filled." Matthew 5:6 NIV*

Pride is the main thing that blinded the Pharisees to the Messiah standing before them, and it is just as debilitating today. For pride hinders us from getting help or being helpful. Pride, taking the form of hypocrisy, will undermine any effort to help people enslaved by addictions. In other instances a subtle form of pride causes us to condemn people who we feel have "brought it on themselves," and then not lift a finger to help them. Instead, let us come together in humility, helping each other to come to the throne of God's grace. It is only there we can truly be of service in combating addictions.

CHAPTER 24

# Doug's Commitment

Doug had been in and out of jail multiple times for possession of drugs and theft to support his drug habit. Each time upon getting out, he would come into my office as part of his court-ordered drug treatment. His visit today followed 30 days in the county jail. Upon entering the exam room, Doug looked at me, his face disconsolate and anxious. He wore a Canucks cap with the brim twisted sideways and a torn Seahawks T-shirt. His jeans were torn and dirty. On his feet he wore scuffed black tennis shoes with loose red laces.

"What happened?" I asked, as I sat down in the exam room.

Doug shrugged and looked down at his shoes. "I guess I am a no good failure."

"I think you have it wrong; the only real failure is failing to try again." I said, in an effort to cheer him up.

"Nice try, Doc, but I've tried a million times to come clean. I just can't do it. My mom's an alcoholic; my dad, last I heard, was doing hard time for drug crimes, and my brother died of an overdose last year. You can't fight genetics. We both know I am hopeless."

"No Doug, you are not hopeless, that is just the drugs talking. But you do sound like someone tired of the battle with addictions," I said trying to judge the seriousness of Doug's despondency.

His head down, Doug continued, "Tired? What I'm tired of is looking in the mirror and seeing my worthless old man staring back. I swore I'd never be like him, but now, I have become what I hate, and hate what I've become."

"That would be tough to live with," I said trying to empathize. But as soon as the words came from my mouth, I tried to clarify, "I don't mean for you to give up on life…"

Doug interrupted, "Actually Doc, I am afraid of dying, but I am getting awful tired of living this way. I want to be clean, but it's just not in me. Even more disgusting is what I've become. You know my only relief is right after I shoot up, and to be honest—that's my only moment of peace—nothing else matters, and I don't care whether I live or die."

Shocked at the dark turn of Doug's thoughts, I blurted out, "Have you ever thought of looking at this mess differently?"

"Huh? What other way is there?" His bleak eyes looked at me.

"Through forgiveness," I replied. "It will take you from where you are, to where God wants you to be."

The notion of forgiveness caught him off guard, and for a moment he had a puzzled look.

"What are you talking about?" he questioned.

"God's forgiveness can set things right between you and Him, and—the result is true peace."

"You mean, just throw around the word 'forgiveness' and everything is made right? Sounds a little hokey," objected Doug. Besides, I've already burned through all the forgiveness I've got coming, just like my dad.

"The power is not in some magical word, nor in whether you feel deserving," I said, "but in the faithfulness of God, who offers forgiveness, and His enduring love that prompts it."

"Look at me, Doc. I'll just mess it up again, so why bother?"

"Forgiveness is not about you promising anything. It's about God telling you He loves you, and how He wants things to be. So God starts you on that road with forgiveness, full and free. Once you receive his forgiveness, then you can give it out to your parents and anyone who has hurt you… even to yourself."

"Yeah, but how good is it when five minutes later, I'm shooting up again?"

"Just as good as the first time," I assured him. "You see

forgiveness is not based on you, but on what Jesus did for you by dying on the cross. He loved you so much He willingly died your death for you, so you could have a new life in Him."

"Isn't God going to tire of me not living up to my end of the bargain?"

"There is no bargain here; it is not tit-for-tat. It is all God's doing. You just need to receive it."

"Right, if only it were that easy, besides how do I know which religion to believe?"

"Because God raised Jesus from the dead. The resurrection of Jesus is proof of his authority and power to forgive and make us clean." I said hoping for Doug to have this joy.

"Same old religious words," Doug moaned. "Nice to hear, but the catch is when it doesn't pan out, and I go back to using, I get blamed for lack of faith, and for not following their rules. There is always something you did, or didn't do with religion."

"There is no catch to forgiveness, you can either accept it, and give thanks, or be stuck holding your bag of guilt and shame."

"See there—laying a guilt trip on me to get me to sign up," said Doug.

"Hold on," I protested. "Weren't you just lamenting that when you look in the mirror you see the shame of your father's face staring back? But in the mirror of God's forgiveness you can look and see what you were meant to be."

"'Meant to be,' almost sounds like a fairy tale." Doug stared at the floor struggling within himself.

I took a deep breath to think, then continued, "Part of drug's deception is to keep you from God's grace by telling you forgiveness has to be earned, or that it is only for decent people. The darkness doesn't want you to know his grace is yours for the asking, because Jesus loves you, and wants to live in you. With such an offer why in the world are you holding back?"

"But, how do I know that it is true?" Doug's voice cracked.

"When Jesus came he did many miracles. They are recorded in the Gospels so that you might believe that Jesus is the Christ, the Son of God, and that by believing you may have LIFE in his name."

"Aw, the Bible is just a bunch of old tales, like every other religion," Doug protested.

"Your addiction has destroyed your life," I said. "What you need is the miracle of God's forgiveness to start with a new life."

"Can I really be different?" Doug asked. "I'm afraid it will end like it always does: I get the shakes and then find a fix."

"How about taking God up on the real fix. Think about this promise:

> *"If we confess our sins, he is faithful and just and will forgive us our sins and purify us from all unrighteousness" 1 John 1:9 NIV*

It says the key we have to turn is confession. When we humbly do this before God, then he forgives and purifies us from our sin.

A glimmer of hope crossed Doug's face, "That's it?

"Yes!" I could hardly keep my composure. "So here is what you commit to: whenever you fail…"

Doug didn't let me finish, "Humbly confess it to God," he mumbled.

"Right! And whenever you wander off?" I posed.

"Humbly confess it, but how do I change?"

"If Jesus has died to bring you forgiveness, He will not leave the miracle half done. He has sent His Spirit to help you live a new life in Him. You just need to trust Him."

Doug's face brightened. In a faint voice he said, "I can do this?"

"Now, let your mind and heart dwell on God's grace and peace to you in Jesus Christ," I said watching joy spread across Doug's face.

"I can do this!" He exclaimed.

**Epilogue**

Doug's life has been added to the great list of miracles Jesus has performed, that we might believe that Jesus is the Christ, the Son of God. It did involve further struggles for Doug, but he kept his commitment to always return and drink in God's grace and peace, and start again new in Jesus.

Most of the New Testament letters start with this blessing: *"Grace and peace to you from God our Father and the Lord Jesus Christ."* This salutation applies to all who seek God's forgiveness and help, it is just a matter of committing to fall before the throne of grace and depend on God to purify you from all unrighteousness. I know Doug would also tell you to rejoice and receive God's forgiveness however many times you need it, for it will never run out. Then, let God's grace and peace in Jesus dwell in you richly—producing the fruit of the Spirit.

**Butterflies From My Tears**

A miraculous gift I have met,
Before my foes a feast is set.
New life arising from Christ's horrid death.
Purest air where I had no breath.
He brings forth food in the driest land,
Hope now gushes from desert sand.
His love squelching the accuser's threats,
Forgiveness silencing my life's regrets.
He wrangles glory from my disgrace,
Victory when I've lost the race.
Bringing butterflies from my tears,
He gives me courage to face my fears.
Hallelujah, Christ's death gives to me,
A wonderful banquet before my enemy.
by Stephen Hufman

God takes our shame and makes us new in Christ.

*"Then God made you alive with Christ, for he forgave all our sins. [14] He canceled the record of the charges against us and took it away by nailing it to the cross. [15] In this way, he disarmed the spiritual rulers and authorities. He shamed them publicly by his victory over them on the cross."*
*Colossians 2:13-15 NIV*

God promises to go with us, preparing a feast where we once had fear.

*"You prepare a feast for me in the presence of my enemies."*
*Psalm 23:5 NIV*

CHAPTER 25

# Dealing with Detoxification

The first hurdle to becoming clean and sober is physical detoxification—getting through the acute physical withdrawal. Current guidelines recommend that detoxification is best done under medical supervision. However, this can be problematic if medical treatment is not available (as is the case in many areas of the country and in 2nd and 3rd world countries). Also, it may be financially out of reach for some people. Another issue is finding a reputable detox unit; unfortunately, there are some programs that are more interested in making money than truly helping. I had one patient who went through a rapid detox unit that promised he would be off opiates in four days. Their method used heavy sedatives to breeze through withdrawal. After paying $18,000, he was sedated for four days to get through withdrawal and left the program dependent on a sedative (Valium) without any after care.

Within days, he had returned to using opiates due to untreated psychological withdrawal (cravings), but was now also taking large amounts of Valium. Unfortunately, sedatives like Valium can also be addicting, and their use with opiates greatly increases the risk of overdose. In this case the patient's choice of a treatment program did not help, but instead added to his problems. Choosing a rehabilitation program should be done with a fair amount of research to insure quality. The standard drug rehabilitation program should have good inpatient psychological and medical care, along with an organized social services program for aftercare and follow up. Keep in mind that secular treatment programs will not provide help for the spiritual side of drug treatment, so the patient will have to take the initiative to set up their own; this is usually accomplished through their support group and family. Always ask rehab programs of their success rate. This is measured by the number who are clean and sober of all drugs after one year, divided by the number who start their program.

Medical supervision can also take the form of an opiate tapering program. This method requires close supervision because the patient will experience mild-to-moderate withdrawal symptoms with each reduction in dose. Craving, and the temptation to abandon the struggle, can become fairly intense and strong, so the patient's support team must be vigilant and active.

There are some patients who do not do well with drug taper and it may be better for them to go "cold turkey" (abruptly stopping the drug). If the patient decides on this course to get over physical withdrawal, they will need to have someone stand watch 24/7 until the physical withdrawal is over. During that time, they will need encouragement from the support group to: maintain drug avoidance, and persevere despite intense craving and strong feelings to give up. If a significant health issue arises, get the patient in for medical evaluation. Obviously, this is a huge responsibility for the support team which is why many elect to do this part of treatment in a rehab facility.

I had one father take his addicted son out camping for a week. It was the worst camping trip ever, but it worked for the acute detoxification phase. However, the family still had to deal with the psychological and spiritual portions of addiction when they returned.

There is one other form of treatment advocated by some, and that is medical maintenance. This involves placing the person on a daily dose of buprenorphine (an opiate substitute) or methadone indefinitely. In this treatment, there is no attempt to get the person off the addictive medication. The benefit is these drugs allow the person to function in a relatively normal fashion. Unfortunately, there are downsides to this treatment that should be considered:

- The person is tethered to the doctor or clinic.

- Moving is difficult because finding a new doctor willing to do maintenance is very hard, and it all has to be worked out in advance of the move to avoid catastrophe.
- Most methadone maintenance clinics only dispense one or two day's worth of pills at a time.
- Patients have told me that tapering and getting off these long-acting drugs (buprenorphine or methadone) is more difficult than coming off short acting opiates.

Being on a maintenance program may reduce the desire to work on the psychological and spiritual aspects of addictions. There is nothing wrong in being in a maintenance program. It does lessen the risk of overdose or contracting a serious illness associated with drug use. But the impetus coming from a desperate need is removed, and the person becomes satisfied with the status quo. Jesus taught in the Parable of the Persistent Widow (Luke 18:1-8) that we should "always pray and never give up." That kind of persistent boldness to ask, knock, and seek (Luke 11:9-12) comes when we realize our desperate need for God's strength and help, and are unwilling to settle for less. Looking at recovery as a means by which God draws the person closer through trials and tribulation adds a spiritual purpose to it all. There will come a day when we will see clearly the spiritual implications of all that has happened. How God used the pain and struggle for His glory. At that moment our earth bound question of "why did You?" will be changed to "Oh Lord, how wonderful!"

*"Some trust in chariots and some in horses,*
*but we trust in the name of the Lord our God." Psalm 20:7 NIV*

*"You, O Lord, keep my lamp burning;*
*My God turns my darkness into light.*
*With your help I can advance against a troop;*

*with my God I can scale a wall." Psalm 18:28-29 NIV*

*"Finally, I urge all:*
*Be joyful in hope, patient in affliction, faithful in prayer."*
*Romans 12:12 NIV*

CHAPTER 26

# Dealing with the Details

*"Blessed is the man whose sin the Lord does not count against him and in whose spirit is no deceit." Psalm 32:2 NIV*

Putting the commitment down in writing is important because later on, during the difficult days of recovery, pulling it out to review will help everyone keep focused, and counter the lies you will tell yourself.

For nicotine addiction the average number of attempts before successful quitting is 9. There is no similar data on narcotic addiction, but we do know many people require multiple attempts, thus success is built on failure and every attempt at stopping gets the person closer to being clean and sober.

Example of a commitment:

I commit to working on my recovery however God wants to do it, for whatever time it takes, daily receiving His grace for my past, and His help for the future. I will strive for honesty in all my dealings, humbly walking with God. To act justly with others and not let my pride get in the way of God's loving mercy, for myself or anyone around me.

*"Then he said to them all: 'If anyone would come after me, he must deny himself and take up his cross daily and follow me.'" Luke 9:23 NIV*

Commitment is important for all followers of Jesus, whether it is in marriage, or work, or recovery from addictions. The reason is that we all face temptation on a daily basis, with the chief temptation being to give up. Therefore, on a daily basis we must renew our commitment and affirm our desire for the LORD to rule over all. Asking Jesus for forgiveness when we wander, and strength to follow Him.

> *"Search me, O God, and know my heart;*
> *test me and know my anxious thoughts.*
> *See if there is any offensive way in me,*
> *and lead me in the way everlasting." Psalm 139:23-24 NIV*

Confession before God, and renewal of trust in him becomes a part of each day, and we commit to do this even when we don't feel like it.

> *"He will keep you strong to the end, so that you will be blameless on the day of our Lord Jesus Christ. God, who has called you into fellowship with his Son Jesus Christ our Lord, is faithful." 1 Corinthians 1:8-9 NIV*

Putting this commitment in writing and signing it helps to affirm the direction the person suffering with addictions wishes to go. Later, this provides an anchor to hold on to when things get rough (and they will get rough).

The next step is to take the pledge and write out a contract that everyone (including family) agrees to follow. It also should be signed, so that everyone is on the same page, and no one has unvoiced expectations.

The contract should include the following:

- If on a drug taper, write out the schedule and who guards the medications (It should be someone trustworthy to handle this responsibility, and not the person taking the prescription).
- Commitment to12-step group attendance (for the

person working on recovery). Specify the number of meetings per week.

- Diligently search for a mentor (not an immediate family member and not someone of the same gender). This accountability partner should have daily contact with the person in recovery.
- Vow to be open and honest (an early warning sign of relapse is when the truth is shaded).
- Make a separate daily schedule of activities that will help avoid triggers (a common trigger is having nothing to do). List the specific triggers that need to be avoided.
- Determine the rules for using the car, phone and Internet (only uses defined in the contract are allowed). Some people will balk at this because they feel it constrains them too much. Almost every drug rehabilitation unit has such rules based on years of experience. Over time, these can be relaxed as the person gains insight and self-control.
- The person should maintain a journal to record and review what he or she is learning.
- List what happens when the contract is not followed. Let the person working on recovery determine the consequences. Make sure these are reasonable, attainable and helpful for recovery. Remember the aim of the consequences is recovery, not punishment. An example might be going to an extra 12-step meeting for 4 weeks, or reformulating the daily schedule making changes that promote sobriety. Breaking the contract must have consequences commensurate with the magnitude of the infraction, but be careful to ensure that the contract will always lead the person to working on their recovery, and not lead to giving up.
- Determine what happens if there is a relapse. If it is of short duration (one day), then determine what went

wrong and correct the contract. Also develop a means to do drug screens to make sure the person continues in recovery (home urine drug screen dip sticks can be purchased on-line). For longer relapses, the whole process must be started again, including the first step of getting the person to humbly acknowledge the addiction and the desperate need to change. The sincerity of this confession can be difficult to assess, since people caught in addiction will lie and say anything. Therefore, rely on actions instead of words. Those who truly desire recovery will be forthcoming about the lies and take responsibility for his or her actions.

- If there is any hint of a problem, do urine drug screening daily.
- The consequences of returning to a life of addiction and its effect on relationships should be laid out clearly. If there are no consequences, then the person will have little reason to restart their recovery. For the family of the addict, this is one of the hardest areas to work out, because it goes against the strong instinct of every parent to keep their child safe by holding them close. For that reason it is covered more thoroughly in the section, "Crossing the Line".

*"Therefore, there is now no condemnation for those who are in Christ Jesus, because through Christ Jesus the law of the Spirit of life set me free from the law of sin and death. For what the law was powerless to do in that it was weakened by the sinful nature, God did by sending his own Son in the likeness of sinful man to be a sin offering. And so he condemned sin in sinful man, in order that the righteous requirements of the law might be fully met in us, who do not live according to the sinful nature but according to the Spirit." Romans 8:1-4 NIV*

CHAPTER 27

# Drawing Boundaries

This section deals with identifying the triggers (internal or external cues that initiate craving the drug) and drawing reasonable boundaries to avoid them. Triggers are like well-worn ruts; if the person falls into one, it is hard to break free before the path leads to relapse. The first step is to draw up a list of triggers and situations which can initiate craving of the drug.

Examples of common triggers:

Places of previous drug use or purchase.

Activities associated with drug use.

People known to use drugs.

Social situations where drugs or alcohol are available .

Objects associated with previous drug use (paraphernalia, credit cards, cell phone, ATMs, empty pill bottles)

Images (movies or pictures depicting drug use).

Music associated with drug use.

The second step is to write out a plan on how to avoid them.

Some triggers are unavoidable. These triggers should also be listed along with a plan of what to do when they occur. These unavoidable triggers will usually require a support person or mentor to help the patient avoid falling further toward relapse. Some other tools to use for fighting triggers are: the use of pre-written letters (see "Rewiring the Brain"), prayers, and memorized Bible verses to remind the patient of the truth. In the case where there is coexisting mental illness, help from a medical professional should be sought as well.

A special situation occurs when the patient in recovery has to deal with acute pain, either from an injury or post surgical pain. Honestly, there is no right answer. Some experts think treating acute pain with narcotics is acceptable and the benefits out-weigh the risks. Unfortunately, I have seen people relapse after being treated with pain medication in the ER. In one case relapse occurred following discharge from the hospital where fentanyl was used as part of the surgical anesthesia. The patient stated that upon awakening from anesthesia he knew something had triggered in him intense craving that he had not had before the surgery. Whatever decision the person makes about narcotics for acute pain, this period should be kept short (~3 days) and requires close support and monitoring. Remember, pain does not kill, but opiates do.

There are medical studies that report opiates make a person more sensitive to pain. What most people report as a light quick pain (e.g. needle stick for drawing blood) a person who has been on opiates will report the pain at a much higher level. The term for this is hyperalgesia. How long this lasts after getting off of opiates is not known. Learning to live with pain is part of the recovery process and may require other modalities to help lessen the hyperalgesia (e.g. Behavior Modification Therapy, hypnosis, or acupuncture).

## Developing Life Skills and Triggers

Another area of potential triggers for drug use is money. All use of money in the past revolved around purchasing drugs. A comprehensive plan for managing money (this includes use of a credit card) is an essential part of rehabilitation and recovery. It should be addressed as part of the contract. Having money can be a trigger and some level of external accountability should be maintained for the first year of recovery. Think of it as learning to budget.

Working is critical to the person's sense of well-being and should be part of the recovery plan. However, there are some jobs that could act as triggers and should be avoided (jobs that allow easy access to drugs or alcohol; such as bar tending, casino work, club bouncer, etc.).

Boundaries

The hardest part of making boundaries is determining appropriate consequences when the lines are crossed. These consequences need to be appropriate to the level of infraction and agreed to in writing by everyone involved, not just the person working on their recovery. The primary goal is recovery, not punishment. If everyone understands that purpose, then the strain on relationships is less, and manipulation is kept to a minimum.

"Crossing the line" occurs on three levels: minor, intermediate, and major. A minor infraction is not likely to lead to relapse but shows disregard for following the contract. These are things like missing a support group meeting, or not checking in with the mentor when running into an unavoidable trigger.

An intermediate infraction has a higher risk and will lead to relapse if not addressed. This encompasses overt disregard of the contract, failing to tell the truth, engaging in an avoidable trigger, or not maintaining contact with their mentor.

A major infraction is use of a drug, or other entity the person is trying to avoid.

Some examples of consequences:

A minor infraction consequence would entail something like an honest discussion of the matter in the support group.

An intermediate infraction consequence would be instituting a daily log of activities and triggers for 5 days, to be reviewed by the mentor. Other consequences could include: loss of independence outside of work, church, and group meetings for a defined period, restricted use of phone and daily review of calls made, and a review of the contract to understand what went wrong and redraw the boundaries.

A major infraction is the most difficult and should be divided into two levels: partial and complete.

Partial relapse (taking the drug only 1 or 2 times) with the consequence being tri-weekly observed urine drug screens, and institution of the intermediate consequence.

Complete relapse should be met with firm insistence to stop using, and all support should be limited to directing the person to stop using. All monetary support is withheld. The person can only return home if there is an agreement to stop using and submit to drug screening to insure compliance. The person also must agree to allow close monitoring until trust is earned back over an extended period.

Theft should be considered complete relapse.

Remember the goal is recovery. So letting consequences slip will usually impede the attainment of becoming clean and sober.

Do not put anything in the contract that all the people involved are not willing to follow, and any subsequent changes must be agreed upon by all.

Mentors are a vital component of the recovery process because they are a source of truth for someone emerging from the influence of drugs. The mentor can cut through the lies of addiction and put forth the truth of God. The mentor encourages and helps during the dark, discouraging times that happen to everyone coming off drugs or alcohol, and is a trusted friend to lean on.

For everyone in recovery, helping others is a way of helping oneself to stay sober. However, you must have a clear assessment of your own boundaries. Otherwise instead of helping, you may be lured back into addictions.

Mentors are usually found in the 12-step group for they

have a basic knowledge of what the addicted person is going

> Mentors should be:
>
> Drug and alcohol free for a prolonged period (3 years).
> The same gender as the person needing help.
> Willing to contact by phone the one being mentored at least once a day.
> Meet face to face once a week.
> Commit to praying daily.
> Be open to calls in the night.

through. A mentor must be careful not to try to take on too many people at one time.

> The Unspoken Consequences:
>
> Every time someone buys an illicit drug, the money goes to an evil empire of sellers, street gangs, smugglers, cartels, and terrorists. The conclusion cannot be avoided that if there were no demand, there would be no money funneling support to these evil entities. How many murders, kidnappings, and wars are happening because of people using drugs is another hideous side to drug abuse.

CHAPTER 28

# Prayer and Fasting

The role of prayer and fasting is very important and often neglected. There are no rules to praying other than: "remember to pray." Time should be set aside to pray daily, with the Bible used both to affirm God's promises, and as a prayer book. Often, I use Bible verses as prayers when my mind won't settle down, or comes under a barrage of anxiety.

*"Even though I walk*
*through the valley of the shadow of death,*
*I will fear no evil,*
*for you are with me." Psalm 23:4 NIV*

Even now as I struggle in the writing of this book, I pray the 23rd Psalm before God, knowing God will lead and go with me.

*"Surely goodness and love will follow me*
*all the days of my life,*
*and I will dwell in the house of the Lord*
*forever." Psalm 23:6 NIV*

Thank you, LORD.

*"Rejoice in the Lord always. I will say it again: Rejoice! Let your gentleness be evident to all. The Lord is near. Do not be anxious about anything, but in everything, by prayer and petition, with thanksgiving, present your requests to God. And the peace of God, which transcends all understanding, will guard your hearts and your minds in Christ Jesus. Finally, brothers, whatever is true, whatever is noble, whatever is right,*

*whatever is pure, whatever is lovely, whatever is admirable—if anything is excellent or praiseworthy—think about such things." Philippians 4:4-8 NIV*

Prayer not only helps change the course of a situation for which one is praying, but also becomes a source of joy for the current moment. It is a blessed assurance that lets you rest and take a deep breath of heavenly air. Other times, one has to specifically ask the Holy Spirit to control ugly fearful thoughts that keep bubbling up from inside. These thoughts make it difficult to pray, but do not be alarmed; this is a normal struggle for everyone. Just continue to pray, for the LORD is listening and wants you to pray on <u>all</u> occasions.

*"And pray in the Spirit on all occasions with all kinds of prayers and requests." Ephesians 6:18 NIV*

The role of fasting, when medically appropriate, is important in breaking the power of addictions, not because fasting somehow gives us leverage with God, but because it reminds us to pray. Fasting causes craving for the food or thing that is being set aside. This intense craving becomes a springboard for prayer. Forcing reliance upon God's strength and not our own. Thus, fasting becomes another way to rewire the brain from the cravings of addiction into something vital to life—communing with God. If you falter at fasting (break the fast) don't condemn yourself, just get up ask for forgiveness and try again…remember this is part of recovery.

A practical but important note about prayer and fasting: If you continually fall asleep while praying, make sure you are getting enough quality sleep. You cannot fight the fight if you are sleep deprived (this includes getting checked for sleep apnea if warranted). Proper nutrition is also important. If your diet lacks vitamins and minerals the body will not function well. Fatigue, a symptom of withdrawal, will be exacerbated by a poor diet. Whether you are working on your recovery or helping someone in recovery these suggestions on prayer and fasting are important spiritual disciplines for everyone.

CHAPTER 29

# Rewiring the Brain

Unfortunately, drugs affect the brain beyond a temporary high. These changes cause the psychological side effects of addiction. One effect is the inability to refuse taking drugs or alcohol when they are accessible. The most glaring example is drug and alcohol consumption during pregnancy.

> In 2014 nearly 32,000 babies were born drug dependent, one every 15 minutes. The problem even has a special name: neonatal abstinence syndrome (NAS). Pediatricians are still unsure how much this prenatal exposure will adversely affect children later in life.

When I asked some of my patients about their substance use during pregnancy, they will often start to cry and say they don't know why they used. At the beginning of their pregnancy they had promised not to take drugs, "It just happened," is the common excuse. This inability to say no is something people without an addiction problem have a hard time understanding—the loss of freedom to choose. Addictions make the brain unable to put off anything you would consider pleasurable. Drugs wire the brain to only choose the easiest and quickest way to get the drug. Thus, lying and cheating become everyday tools to get drugs. Right and wrong no longer have any say in decisions the person makes.

Human nature has this tendency for instant gratification; like a person trying to lose weight denying himself chocolate cake, resistance is difficult. Unfortunately, with drugs and alcohol, the craving is a hundred times worse. Addictions make it mentally impossible to wait. The drug becomes the solution to every problem, to every discomfort. It becomes the sole key to feeling normal. Some will see this as just another excuse to continue using drugs, but I bring it up because this damage to the brain is real, and it has to be addressed to achieve long-term recovery.

> *"Trust in the Lord with all your heart*
> *and lean not on your own understanding;*
> *in all your ways acknowledge him,*
> *and he will make your paths straight.*
> *Do not be wise in your own eyes;*
> *fear the Lord and shun evil.*
> *This will bring health to your body*
> *and nourishment to your bones."*
> *Proverbs 3:5-8 NIV*

There are two aspects to the hard work of rewiring the brain. The first is to bring in outside help: the addict needs a mentor whom they trust. The mentor speaks truth to counter the lies and thoughts of an addicted brain and supply strength until the intense craving subsides. The second aspect is trying to reprogram the brain and bring healing to the thought processes. I call this reprograming process "Letters from the heart to the mind about addictions." The point of these exercises is not to tell people how they should think, but to get them to work on how they will change their thinking. Carefully writing out thoughts and reasons for sobriety helps the person use other areas of the brain to take on a stronger role and squash cravings with truth. This assists the brain in rediscovering what sober thinking is like and reinforces how their previous thoughts and cravings got them into trouble. In doing this exercise, I ask the patient not to rant or yell at themselves but to write in a manner that would persuade them to take the path toward sobriety.

**Suggested topics for letters to the brain from the heart:**

Write a letter declaring why you desperately need to stop using. It is not crying over what has happened, but laying out the horrible life of addiction and consequences that will occur if you do not quit. End with a statement of hope, of purpose, and of God's ultimate goal. This letter becomes a personal statement of what life is truly about.

Make a list of the promises of God and add to them as you discover more in the Bible. The goal is to memorize these verses, so they can become anchors to your soul when drugs try to whipsaw your mind with lies and accusations.

**Some examples of memory verses:**

*"The Lord will fight for you; you need only to be still." Exodus 14:14 NIV*

*"The Lord himself goes before you and will be with you; he will never leave you nor forsake you. Do not be afraid; do not be discouraged." Deuteronomy 31:8 NIV*

*"He gives strength to the weary and increases the power of the weak. Even youths grow tired and weary, and young men stumble and fall; but those who hope in the Lord will renew their strength. They will soar on wings like eagles; they will run and not grow weary, they will walk and not be faint." Isaiah 40:29-31 NIV*

*"So do not fear, for I am with you; do not be dismayed, for I am your God. I will strengthen you and help you; I will uphold you with my righteous right hand." Isaiah 41:10 NIV*

*"For God so loved the world that he gave his one and only Son, that whoever believes in him shall not perish but have eternal life. For God did not send his Son into the world to condemn*

*the world, but to save the world through him." John 3:16-17 NIV*

*"Submit yourselves, then, to God. Resist the devil, and he will flee from you." James 4:7 NIV*

*"If we confess our sins, he is faithful and just and will forgive us our sins and purify us from all unrighteousness." 1 John 1:9 NIV*

**Other suggestions for letters:**

Write a letter to yourself for the moment before you took your first drug. Recall what you were thinking, the peer pressure, and point out the lies. Gently but convincingly state the truth. State the aftermath of that terrible day and list all the problems you never saw coming. Share these thoughts with your mentor and support group so all may benefit.

Write a letter to yourself describing your enslavement. Start with what makes your addiction so attractive and then unveil the dark side. Warn yourself and others how to avoid this path. What would you have told yourself to prevent that first step into addictions?

Write a letter to yourself in the moments just before you relapse. Point out what lines you crossed that allowed you to come to that point. What excuses did you tell yourself? What could you have done or thought to change your course? Remember, your brain lacks the ability to say no.

Write out a practical plan for dealing with cravings that involves focusing on healthy and good activities.

Cultivating impulse control:

Ask God to produce the fruit of the Spirit (Galatians 5:22-23).

Memorize scripture that promises good things (Romans 8:37-39; Philippians 4:4-7) then repeat it when you feel things going the wrong direction. Remember Bible verses are truth to combat the lies, not some magic spell. Therefore, keep reviewing and praying the verses until the craving passes. If it just won't stop, call your mentor.

Write a letter of encouragement to someone who becomes tired of fighting against addiction (they feel like giving up). Pretend you are their mentor. What would you tell them? Write a letter from the last day of your life. Speak to what is important from that perspective.

Write a letter to your children that will show them how to avoid your mistakes. Give them guidance on how they should live.

Write to someone you have hurt. Tell them what you did and why it was wrong. Ask for forgiveness and tell them what you have learned. Caution, this letter is not to be shared unless you are sure the sharing will not cause further harm.

Write to someone who has hurt you. Tell them what they did and how it hurt you. Tell them how it should have been. Discuss what forgiveness means to them, to you, and to God.

Write out Celebrate Recovery's Eight Principles and add what each Bible verse means to you personally. https://www.

celebraterecovery.com/resources/cr-tools/8principles

**Celebrate Recovery's Eight Recovery Principles:**
**The Road to Recovery Based on the Beatitudes**

Realize I'm not God; I admit that I am powerless to control my tendency to do the wrong thing and that my life is unmanageable. (Step 1)

*"Happy are those who know that they are spiritually poor." Matthew 5:3a TEV*

Earnestly believe that God exists, that I matter to Him and that He has the power to help me recover. (Step 2)

*"Happy are those who mourn, for they shall be comforted." Matthew 5:4 TEV*

Consciously choose to commit all my life and will to Christ's care and control. (Step 3)

*"Happy are the meek." Matthew 5:5a TEV*

Openly examine and confess my faults to myself, to God, and to someone I trust. (Steps 4 and 5)

*"Happy are the pure in heart." Matthew 5:8a TEV*

Voluntarily submit to any and all changes God wants to make in my life and humbly ask Him to remove my character defects. (Steps 6 and 7)

*"Happy are those whose greatest desire is to do what God requires" Matthew 5:6a TEV*

Evaluate all my relationships. Offer forgiveness to those who have hurt me and make amends for harm I've done to others when possible, except when to do so would harm them or others. (Steps 8 and 9)

*"Happy are the merciful." Matthew 5:7a TEV; "Happy are the peacemakers" Matthew 5:9 TEV*

Reserve a daily time with God for self-examination, Bible reading, and prayer in order to know God and His will for my life and to gain the power to follow His will. (Steps 10 and 11)

Yield myself to God to be used to bring this Good News to others, both by my example and my words. (Step 12)

*"Happy are those who are persecuted because they do what God requires." Matthew 5:10 TEV*

These letters are not intended to be sent. They are simply a means to work at rewiring thinking and perception. When the author of the letters feels shaky about staying clean, he can pull out the letters and read them to remind himself of correct thinking and not get fooled by the lies of addiction.

**Negative Thought Cycles**

Negative thought cycles occur in most people, but in addiction they can lead to relapse or even worse--suicidal feelings. The strength and persistence of negative thoughts vary from person to person usually taking the form of an accusatory inner voice stoking the fire of guilt, shame and worthlessness. Combating these negative thoughts involves three steps:

**Step one:** Recognition.

It is amazing how often we can ruminate over some negative event and not realize it until we are stuck in a deepening depression. Labeling our thoughts as negative begins the process of isolating them and stopping the cycle.

Negative thoughts usually fall into four groups:

1) Dwelling on a failure or wrong that you cannot release, or avoid thinking about.

2) Feelings of inadequacy.

3) Catastrophe: Making an interaction or minor event into a something much worse.

4) Blaming yourself for anything that doesn't go as expected.

**Step two:** Getting off the negative thought merry-go-round.

1) Ask God for forgiveness and claim 1 John 1:9 — "If we confess our sins He is faithful and just to forgive our sins and cleanse us from all unrighteousness." Do not fret if you still feel guilt and shame for your actions. That is normal, but you can reject it each time it pops up. Remember, we receive righteousness by faith not by feeling. For in the gospel, a righteousness from God is revealed, a righteousness that is by faith from first to last, just as it is written: "The righteous will live by faith." Romans 1:17

2) Write down all that you are grateful for (count your blessings, name them one by one).

3) Review how God has brought you through past trials and praise Him for it.

4) Write down all the things that causing negative thoughts.

5) Affirm that God is in control of all things and thank him for his love and faithfulness.

**Step three:**

Repeat the steps one and two until you are full of God's grace and peace.

If you are stuck in a negative thought cycle or depression, then seek out a professional counselor for help. There is no shame in this for the truth of being God's child is accurate. You just need further help in finding how to rest in it.

CHAPTER 30

# Codependency

At 12-step meetings people will often mention codependency as something they struggle with. Understanding what it is and how it works is half the battle in straightening out its entanglement.

"Co-" a Latin prefix meaning together used with the word dependence speaks to a relationship that depends on someone or something for the persons well being. We were created to be dependent on God and His love. Things get twisted when we try to fill our need for God with someone or something else. To expect someone to fill God's role in life is not going to work and leads to codependency. An example is a parent who won't let their child grow up because they are afraid of being alone. For many codependency starts with dysfunctional relationships learned as a child in a family dominated by manipulation and selfishness rather than reflecting God's loving character. Codependency also happens as a consequence of alcohol and drug abuse where the substance takes the place of God.

As the word codependency implies, Codependence is the worship and dependence upon something or someone other than God alone. No matter what other god you choose, be it yourself, your family, drugs, or things, the result is the same—you will be enslaved to what you worship, and that misplaced worship will be toxic to yourself and everyone around you.

Some people who are caught in codependence fell into it because they were born into dysfunctional families. Unfortunately, they have learned dysfunctional ways to give and receive love (some of it is not really love just trying to fill emotional needs in the wrong way). My hope is that this discussion will help people understand how complete dependence upon God and drawing close to Him for all our needs, allows other relationships to flourish as God intended. By letting go of depending on others to meet what only the love of God can fill, you can begin to love others untethered by what you get out of it. Building relationships based on the pattern of God's love for us in Jesus.

I first met Rhonda when she came in for prenatal care late in her pregnancy. She had just moved to our small town from another state and needed to establish care.

"So why did you move here so late in your pregnancy?" I said scanning the medical records she brought with her.

She paused to consider her words then shrugged her shoulders, "It's a long story, are you sure you want to hear it?"

"I want to hear whatever you're willing to tell me."

"Aunt Betty insisted I come to get away from my boyfriend, Chris."

"Is he the father?" I said watching her shift uneasy in the chair.

"Uh-huh."

"Why did your aunt think you should get away from him?"

"He hit me, but just once, and only because he had been drinking again."

"So, Chris has a drinking problem?"

"He promised me he'd stop. That's the only way I would go out with him."

"But, he didn't stop did he?" I suggested.

"No, he did stop, it was just the stress of the pregnancy that made him drink. It's really my fault. He wanted me to get an abortion, but I wouldn't 'cause it goes against my beliefs."

"So Chris doesn't have the same beliefs as you?"

"Oh, Chris is really nice," Rhonda seemed to brighten. "I know he is close to 'cepting Jesus, but this whole thing set him back a bit. I told him we couldn't get married unless he became a believer. I know God has great things in store for Chris."

"What do your parents think about your pregnancy with Chris?"

"My mom just wants me to be happy I guess. We don't talk much."

"And your dad?"

Sadness came over Rhonda, "He left us five years ago… Mom got tired of his drinking. I tried to get him to stop, but… he left instead. He has a new family now. They take up all of his time."

"That must hurt," I said.

"Yeah it did, but I have Chris now."

"With all you have been through have you considered seeing a counselor."

"What for?" Rhonda said a little defensive.

"You may have some unresolved issues with your dad that could be affecting things now. Have you ever heard of codependency?"

"Has my aunt been talking to you?"

"No, I can't discuss with anyone what goes on here without your permission."

"Well, she wants me to see a counselor, too. I think to try to keep me from going back to Chris. Aunt Betty thinks I'm using Chris as a substitute for my dad."

"Are you?"

"No, I love Chris and he needs me."

"I don't think it would hurt to talk with a counselor at least once, then you can decide if it's worthwhile."

"I'll think about it," Rhonda replied.

Over the next six weeks the topic never came up again.

Rhonda had a long hard labor and delivery, her aunt stayed with her through the whole ordeal. But what really hurt Rhonda was that Chris never called her. He ended up getting another girlfriend and dumping Rhonda and baby Christopher. Because of this Rhonda finally saw a counselor, and started working through all the pent-up hurt. She learned how it affected every relationship even her relationship with God. The other thing that made Rhonda work at her codependency became helping her son overcome his own rejection by his father and not be trapped into repeating the cycle of codependency.

~

In the Gospel of John, Jesus declares that He is totally dependent on God the Father (a relationship of dependence):

> *"I tell you the truth, the Son can do nothing by himself; he can do only what he sees his Father doing because whatever the Father does the Son also does. For the Father loves the Son and shows him all he does." John 5:19-20 NIV*

This dependence is voluntary, total and based on love. Jesus turns and invites us to join him in this wonderful intimacy with God.

> *"As the Father has loved me, so have I loved you. Now remain in my love. If you obey my commands, you will remain in my love, just as I have obeyed my Father's commands and remain in his love.... My command is this: Love each other as I have loved you." John 15:9-12 NIV*

Codependency is trying to serve and love another person (or thing) with a devotion and dependence that should only be given to God. The rub is you cannot be totally dependent upon God (serving and loving Him above all else), and at the same time trying to serve and love someone else coequal with God. In fact, Jesus tells us this will not work:

> *"No one can serve two masters. Either he will hate the one and*

*love the other, or he will be devoted to the one and despise the other. You cannot serve both God and Money." Matthew 6:24 NIV*

And later Jesus states:

*"Anyone who loves his father or mother more than me is not worthy of me; anyone who loves his son or daughter more than me is not worthy of me; and anyone who does not take his cross and follow me is not worthy of me. Whoever finds his life will lose it, and whoever loses his life for my sake will find it." Matthew 10:37-39 NIV*

This last verse makes it clear that trying to find your life in anything besides Jesus will turn into a terrible loss. It is that way with codependency. It tries to elevate a relationship with someone on par, or greater than, our complete reliance upon God. In addictions, this begins when the drug commands subservience to it rather than to God.

The temptations of Jesus centered on this very issue of total subservience to God. In the first temptation, Satan challenged Jesus to move out from dependence upon God. "You're hungry, use your power to make these stones into bread," Satan wanted Jesus to act independently from God to resolve his hunger. Jesus responded, "Man does not live on bread alone, but on every word that comes from the mouth of God."

The second temptation involved Jesus forcing God to act.

*Then the devil took him to the holy city and had him stand on the highest point of the temple. "If you are the Son of God," he said, "throw yourself down. For it is written: 'He will command his angels concerning you, and they will lift you up in their hands, so that you will not strike your foot against a stone.'" Matthew 4:5-6 NIV*

This is a manipulation, a tool people use to control others for their own purpose. Jesus responds: "*Do not put the Lord your God to the test.*"

The final temptation revolved around the issue of control. Jesus would get complete control of everything if He would bow and worship Satan along with God. Jesus answered, "*Worship the Lord your God, and serve him only.*"

Competing for control is often the underlying issue in codependent relationships. Any relationship where you are trying to take God's place or push others into God's role, will only end in disappointment and dysfunction.

CHAPTER 31

# Anxiety and Addictions

Anxiety is common in life and often arises when trying to free oneself from addictions. You have to have a plan for dealing with anxiety in recovery because in the past, the drug is what you used to calm anxiety. You will need to learn a safe and clean way of getting through nervousness so the anxiety-addiction loop can be broken. Finding a professional counselor to work with you on this can be helpful.

If you are doing a drug taper, there will be anxiety with each drop in medication. If you are clean and off drugs, anxiety can be a trigger to relapse. Anticipating this in life is important for planning strategies to avoid falling back into drug use. The task is to develop healthy ways of handling anxiety. Do not fall into the trap of using tranquilizers (e.g. Valium); this is trading addictions and does nothing to generate internal methods of dealing with anxiety.

**Practical ideas for dealing with anxiety:**

Read and pray the Twenty-third Psalm.

Exercise to the point of exhaustion; relief starts when you are too tired to think of anything but being out of breath. It uses up the adrenaline surge from anxiety and releases calming parasympathetic neuro-chemicals.

Review God's promises (this requires a prepared list of verses that you repeat out loud). After each promise repeat:

*"Give thanks to the Lord, for he is good. His love endures forever."*

Write all the things for which you are grateful (count your blessings).

When the anxiety is about past wrongs, repeat:

> *"As far as the East is from the West, so far has he removed our transgressions from us." Psalm 103:12*

Find other verses that declare how God has removed your past mistakes.

Identify the fears that are making you anxious. Write them down and pray over them. Then crumple the paper and throw them away. Repeat:

> *"The name of the LORD is a strong tower; the righteous run to it and they are safe." Proverbs 18:10 NIV*

Practice abdominal breathing (inhale expanding your stomach not the chest) for 4 counts, hold for 2 counts, exhale over 4 counts, hold for 2 counts, repeat. As you do this, let your entire body deflate with each exhalation.

Write out all the negative self-talks that run through your mind (see chapter on "Negative Thought Cycles"), then write out Bible verses that reveal God's truth about you. An example of a negative self-talk: "I can't do this, what's the use of trying anymore?" Bible verse:

> *"For it is by grace you have been saved, through faith—and this not from yourselves, it is the gift of God— not by works, so that no one can boast. For we are God's workmanship, created in Christ Jesus to do good works, which God prepared in advance for us to do." Ephesians 2:8-10 NIV*

Some anxiety has its roots in previous experiences or trauma (PTSD), which requires further processing. If PTSD triggers suicidal thoughts, or of causing harm to anyone, then get immediate help. This can be done through a professional counselor, or call National Suicide Prevention Lifeline (1-800-273-8255).

To work on taming PTSD, start by writing a narrative of

the trauma, including details like smells, sounds, feelings, and thoughts. The first writing will most likely not capture all of the emotion, so keep working at it. This revisiting of a traumatic experience may seem scary. These are thoughts we want to bury not dig up, but if you stick with it, the events will lose their power over you. The words you write will give you a handle on the event, shedding light on this dark place. It is like turning the light on in the closet; the shapes and scary feelings shrink back to old clothes on hangers. The event will always be painful but will not produce as much fearful reaction. With less guilt and self-blame, the anxiety and physical symptoms will recede. Picture yourself laying the burden down at the Cross of Christ: all the guilt, the shame and fear now belongs to Jesus.

*"Come to me, all you who are weary and burdened, and I will give you rest. Take my yoke upon you and learn from me, for I am gentle and humble in heart, and you will find rest for your souls. For my yoke is easy and my burden is light." Matthew 11: 28-30 NIV*

Remember to pray and let others pray with you.

*"Do not be anxious about anything, but in everything, by prayer and petition, with thanksgiving, present your requests to God. And the peace of God, which transcends all understanding, will guard your hearts and your minds in Christ Jesus." Philippians 4:6-7 NIV*

At some point, if you like, you can share the anxiety producing story with others who are close to you. The intent of this is not to drum up sympathy, but it is to let the pain go, and sharing does that. When you share your story with someone you trust, it will build the relationship, allowing them to feel closer to you. "A sorrow shared is half the sorrow. A joy shared is twice the joy" (Scandinavian proverb).

Have a fall-back plan for times when the emotions become overwhelming. For most people, this occurs at least once in their recovery. First, decide what are the early signs that this is happening, like rumination that doesn't stop after a minute or two. Next, form a list of people willing to talk to you over the phone or in person. Their role is to listen, then pray, then review Bible verses until there is easing of the anxiety (caution: reviewing verses should be about reassurance not about "come on buck up"). This personal contact is essential to reminding the patient of what is true and real until things calm down. Also, it's important to have someone there to prevent the person from using drugs to treat the anxiety. (A word to this friend: listen, listen, listen).

CHAPTER 32

# Family Contract

It is easy for people to fall into enabling because families and friends want to help. The problem is how to help without becoming an impediment to recovery through enabling. There is no exact formula for avoiding enabling, because each family situation is different, but there are some definite directives one should follow in drawing up a family contract.

Do what you already know is the right thing to do before God, even when you feel it is in an unrelated matter. Things like being truthful in all your ways and not being involved with anything illegal or immoral. Treat each other with kindness and love. Do not let the sun go down on your anger. Forgive each other. Be intentional about following Jesus in all your ways. Obviously, this will not be easy, but if you want your son or daughter to recognize their need for God, you must recognize your own, and seek the Lord's help.

Do not allow drugs of abuse in the house by anyone (this includes alcohol and marijuana).

Keep all prescription drugs locked up.

Remember that the goal is to help the person become clean and sober; therefore, do not permit any activity that does not move in that direction. (See section on triggers "Drawing Your Boundaries")

If the family member struggling with addictions is living at home, they must be involved in rehabilitation.

Do not let the strain of addiction destroy family relationships among other family members. This will require work and vigilance on everyone's part, especially between spouses.

Work at communication, talk things over, be transparent with your spouse.

Pray together.

Work at loving each other.

*Love is patient and kind. Love is not jealous or boastful or proud or rude. It does not demand its own way. It is not irritable, and it keeps no record of being wronged. It does not rejoice about injustice but rejoices whenever the truth wins out. Love never gives up, never loses faith, is always hopeful, and endures through every circumstance. 1 Corinthians 13:4-7 NLT*

SECTION 8

# Final Need

I have a confession to make. I am made of the same stuff as any person addicted to drugs, or pornography, or gambling, or video games, and so is everyone on the planet. We are unable to choose correctly, we cannot maintain any self-discipline, we are subject to mental illness, eating disorders, social anxiety, and enslaving fears. We manipulate and are easily manipulated; we lie and cheat and hide our true selves behind a facade of looking normal. Always being afraid of the day when we will be discovered and the truth revealed. My confession is I am in desperate need of God's help. I don't deserve it, I can't earn it, and my need is not "just this once," but stretches out to every breath from my first cry, to my last sigh. I need forgiveness and ongoing help from Jesus. But that is just where God wants us--hungering and thirsting for Him. Then, as we trust Him in all things, He will bring about the miracle we seek.

> *"Come to me, all you who are weary and burdened, and I will give you rest. Take my yoke upon you and learn from me, for I am gentle and humble in heart, and you will find rest for your souls. For my yoke is easy and my burden is light." - Jesus Matthew 11:28-30 NIV*

Jesus wants to help us. He invites us to come to him. So that no matter where we are in recovery, or this earthly life, we can marvel with the Psalmist and say:

> *"You hem me in—behind and before;*
> *You have laid your hand upon me.*
> *Such knowledge is too wonderful for me,*
> *too lofty for me to attain.*

*Where can I go from your Spirit?*
*Where can I flee from your presence?*
*If I go up to the heavens, you are there;*
*if I make my bed in the depths, you are there.*
*If I rise on the wings of the dawn,*
*if I settle on the far side of the sea,*
*even there your hand will guide me,*
*your right hand will hold me fast."*
*Psalm 139:5-10 NIV*

I am thankful for life, but what fills me with unspeakable joy is the wonderful grace of Jesus in my life now and forever. A grace from God not of my own making, nor mine for breaking. Grace allows me in this moment, regardless of my past, to rest in Jesus. I can fellowship with God now, and know He will go with me, hold on to me, give me purpose, and see me home to be with him forever.

Our desperate need is to humbly bow before Jesus and let Him work in our lives. Not just for recovery from our addictions, but to mold us into the glorious person He has planned. Little do we know of all the amazing things God wants to bring forth in and through us. What God asks of us is to show up audaciously before the throne of grace and seek him. Too often we let negative thoughts turn us away from praying. Jesus taught about approaching the throne of God when we do not feel like it (for whatever reason):

*"But I tell you this—though he won't do it for friendship's sake, if you keep knocking long enough, he will get up and give you whatever you need because of your shameless persistence. And so I tell you, keep on asking, and you will receive what you ask for. Keep on seeking, and you will find. Keep on knocking, and the door will be opened to you." Luke 11:8-9 NLT*

Shameless persistence?

Shameless defined: Acting without shame, characterized by or showing lack of shame where one should have shame. To abandon any sense of decorum.

Shameless persistence is ignoring all the reasons you shouldn't or can't ask God, and throw yourself at the feet of Jesus again and again. Shameless is the women who being unclean from years of bleeding crawled in the dirt to touch Jesus' cloak (Luke 8:43-48). Shameless is the thief on the cross who after heaping insults upon Jesus, turned and asked to be remembered when Jesus came into His kingdom (Luke 23:42).

Jesus teaches us about prayer in Luke 11. He tells us to be shameless and persistent in asking, seeking, and knocking. This is an encouragement to be outrageously bold in prayer regardless of our worthiness.

Whatever reason your mind puts up for why you can't seek God's mercy, or that it is the wrong time to knock at His door, cast aside all pride and be shameless in prayer. Then keep doing it with reckless abandon until you receive help from God to live for Him.

When you are bored, looking in the wrong places for excitement—pray for joy.

When you are too tired to care—pray for strength.

When you have betrayed God—pray for redemption.

When you are angry and can't forgive—pray for mercy.

When you have squandered every opportunity—pray for help.

When you are dying from guilt—pray for forgiveness and grace to live.

Remember, there is no occasion or circumstance that can separate you from the love of God, so pray with shameless persistence.

*"Let us then approach the throne of grace with confidence, so*

*that we may receive mercy and find grace to help us in our time of need." Hebrews 4:16 NIV*

When I am shamelessly persistent in prayer and confident in approaching the throne of grace, I can take my focus off me and put it wholly upon Jesus… I just need to show up totally dependent on Him.

I would like to add a 13$^{th}$ step to the 12-step program. It is a step for all of us on this journey called life. Step 13: rest and walk in the grace and peace of Jesus Christ. This means that anyone who belongs to Christ can rest in the fact that they are a new person. In God's eyes the old life with all its wrongs and hurts has been wiped away and a new life has begun! (2 Corinthians 5:17)

You may think that takes care of my past, but what of my future mess-ups?

*"Being confident of this, that he who began a good work in you will carry it on to completion until the day of Christ Jesus." Philippians 1:6 NIV*

Therefore, since we have been made right in God's sight by faith, we have peace with God because of what Jesus Christ our Lord has done for us. In Christ we are brought into a place of undeserved privilege before God where we now stand as His children. This means with confidence and joy we can look forward to sharing God's glory.

*We can rejoice, too, when we run into problems and trials, for we know that they help us develop endurance. And endurance develops strength of character, and character strengthens our confident hope of salvation. And this hope will not lead to disappointment. For we know how dearly God loves us because he has given us the Holy Spirit to fill our hearts with his love." Romans 5:1-5 NLT*

So I end with the salutation Paul used in his letters to fellow believers… Grace, mercy, and peace to you from God our Father, and the Lord Jesus Christ.

Amen.

# Resources

To learn more about codependency:

Hemfelt, R., Minirth, F., & Meier, P. (2003). *Love Is a Choice: The Definitive Book on Letting Go of Unhealthy Relationships.* Nashville, Tennessee: Thomas Nelson, Inc.

Lancer, D. (2015). *Codendency for Dummies, 2nd Edition.* Hoboken, New Jersey: John Wiley & Sons, Inc.

**Resources for Addictions and Codependency**

Alcoholics Anonymous

https://www.aa.org/

Overcomers Outreach

http://www.overcomersoutreach.org/

Celebrate Recovery

http://www.celebraterecovery.com/

Emotions Anonymous

http://emotionsanonymous.org/

Narcotics Anonymous

https://www.na.org/

Codependents Anonymous

http://coda.org/

National Association for Children of Alcoholics

https://nacoa.org/

Adult Children of Alcoholics

http://www.adultchildren.org/

Incest Survivors Anonymous

http://www.siawso.org/

Al-Anon

http://al-anon.org/

# References

Introduction, page iii
(2015). Ilicit Drug Use. Retreived from https://www.drugabuse.gov/publications/drugfacts/nationwide-trends

Chapter 1, page 3
Cheatle, M. & Comer, D. and others (2014). Treating Pain in Addicted Patients: Recommendations from and Expert Panel. Retrieved from https://www.ncbi.nlm.nih.gov/pmc/articles/PMC3996998/

Chapter 7, page 47a
Hasin, D. S. & O'Brien, C. P. and others (2013). DSM-5 Criteria for Substance Use Disorders. Retrieved from https://www.ncbi.nlm.nih.gov/pmc/articles/PMC3767415/

Chapter 7, page 47b
Murthy, V. H. (2016). Facing Addiction in America - Surgeon General's Report on Alcohol, Drugs, and Health. Retrieved from https://addiction.surgeongeneral.gov/sites/default/files/surgeon-generals-report.pdf

Chapter 9, page 58
CDC. Impaired Driving: Get the Facts. Retrieved from https://www.cdc.gov/motorvehiclesafety/impaired_driving/impaired-drv_factsheet.html

Chapter 9, page 59
NIH. Priciples of Adolescent Substance Use Disorder Treatment. Retrieved from https://www.drugabuse.gov/publications/principles-adolescent-substance-use-disorder-treatment-research-based-guide/frequently-asked-questions/it-possible-teens-to-become-addicted-to-marijuana